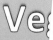 

# Ve

| | | |
|---|---|---|
| 1- Amaranth Leaves | 2-Arrowroot | 3-Artichoke |
| 4-Arugula | 5-Asparagus | 6-Bamboo Shoots |
| 7-Beans (Green) | 8-Beets | 9-Belgian Endive |
| 10-Bitter Melon | 11-Bok Choy | 12-Broadbeans |
| 13-Broccoli | 14-Broccoli Rabe | 15-Brussel Sprouts |
| 16-Cabbage (Green) | 17-Cabbage, Red | 18-Carrot |
| 19-Cassava (Yuca Root) | 20-Cauliflower | 21-Celeriac |
| 22-Celery | 23-Chayote | 24-Chicory |
| 25-Collards | 26-Corn | 27-Crookneck |
| 28-Cucumber | 29-Daikon | 30-Dandelion Greens |
| 31-Edamame, Soybeans | 32-Eggplant | 33-Fennel |
| 34-Fiddleheads | 35-Ginger Root | 36-Horseradish |
| 37-Jicama | 38-Kale | 39-Kohlrabi |
| 40-Leeks | 41-Lettuce, Iceberg | 42-Lettuce, Leaf |
| 43-Lettuce, Romaine | 44-Mushrooms | 45-Mustard Greens |
| 46-Okra | 47-Onion (Red) | 48-Onions |
| 49-Parsnip | 50-Peas, Green | 51-Pepper, Green |
| 52-Pepper, Sweet Red | 53-Potato, Red | 54-Potato, White |
| 55-Potato, Yellow | 56-Pumpkin | 57-Radicchio |
| 58-Radishes | 59-Rutabaga | 60-Salsify |
| 61-Shallots | 62-Snow Peas | 63-Sorrel (Dock) |
| 64-Spaghetti Squash | 65-Spinach | 66-Squash, Butternut |
| 67-Sugar Snap Peas | 68-Sweet Potato | 69-Swiss Chard |
| 70-Tomatillo | 71-Tomato | 72-Turnip |

# *Amaranth leaves*

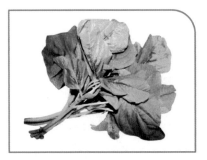

### How to store?

Keep refrigerated in a plastic bag. Use within one week.

### Benefits:

- Antioxydant agent
- Inprove digestion
- Improve vision
- Helps with hair loss
- Prevents Atherosclerosis

## NUTRITIONAL RATIO

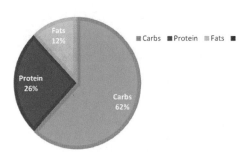

■ Carbs  ■ Protein  ■ Fats  ■

### Nutrition Values for 100g

**Energy:** 23 Kcal

**Carbohydrate:** 4.02 g

**Protein:** 2.46 g

**Total fat:** 0.33 g

**Dietary fiber:** 2.2 g

| Vitamin | Value | RDA % |
|---|---|---|
| Vitamin A | 2917 IU | 97% |
| Vitamin C | 43.3 mg | 70.5% |
| Vitamin K | 1140 µg | 950% |
| Folates | 85 µg | 21% |
| Niancin | 0.658 mg | 4% |
| Pantothenic acid | 0.065 mg | 1% |
| Pyridoxine | 0.192 mg | 15% |
| Riboflavin | 0.158 mg | 12% |
| Thiamin | 0..027 mg | 2% |

| Minerals | Value | RDA% |
|---|---|---|
| Calcium | 215 mg | 21.5% |
| Copper | 0.162 mg | 18% |
| Iron | 2.32 mg | 29% |
| Magnesium | 55 mg | 14% |
| Manganese | 0.885 mg | 38% |
| Phosphorus | 50 mg | 7% |
| Zinc | 0.90 mg | 8% |

# *Arrowroot*

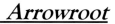

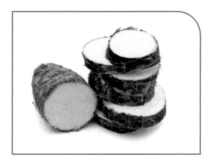

## How to store?

Store for up to 2 weeks in a plastic bag in the fridge.

## Benefits:

- Aids Digestion
- Beneficial In Pregnancy
- Improve brain functioning
- strengthen the heart
- Improve kidney health

## NUTRITIONAL RATIO

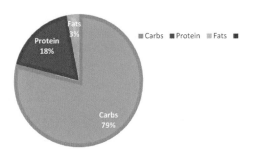

### Nutrition Values for 100g

**Energy:** 65 Kcal

**Carbohydrate:** 13.39 g

**Protein:** 4.24 g

**Total fat:** 0.20 g

**Dietary fiber:** 1.3 g

| Vitamin | Value | RDA % |
|---|---|---|
| Vitamin A | 19 IU | 1% |
| Vitamin C | 1.9 mg | 3% |
| Folates | 338 µg | 84% |
| Niancin | 1.693 mg | 10.5% |
| Pyridoxine | 0.266 mg | 20% |
| Riboflavin | 0.059 mg | 4.5% |
| Thiamin | 0.143 mg | 12% |

| Minerals | Value | RDA% |
|---|---|---|
| Calcium | 6 mg | 0.6% |
| Copper | 0.121 mg | 13.5% |
| Iron | 2.22 mg | 28% |
| Magnesium | 25 mg | 6% |
| Manganese | 0.174 mg | 7.5% |
| Phosphorus | 98 mg | 14% |
| Selenium | 0.7 µg | 1% |
| Zinc | 0.63 mg | 6% |

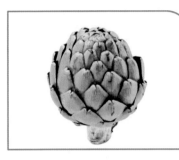

# *Artichoke*

### How to store?

Cover and refrigerate for up to 1 week.

### Benefits:

- Bowels cleaner
- Improve heart health
- Inprove mental health
- Strong anti-cancer
- Improve liver and gallbladder function

## NUTRITIONAL RATIO

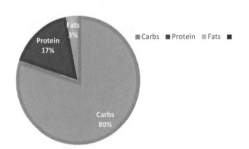

■ Carbs ■ Protein ■ Fats ■

## Nutrition Values for 100g

**Energy:** 47 Kcal

**Carbohydrate:** 10.51 g

**Protein:** 3.27 g

**Total fat:** 0.15 g

**Dietary fiber:** 5.4 g

| Vitamin | Value | RDA % |
|---|---|---|
| Vitamin A | 13 IU | 0.5% |
| Vitamin C | 11.7 mg | 20% |
| Vitamin E | 0.19 mg | 1% |
| Vitamin K | 14.8 µg | 12% |
| Folates | 68 µg | 17% |
| Niancin | 1.046 mg | 6.5% |
| Pantothenic acid | 0.338 mg | 7% |
| Pyridoxine | 0.166 mg | 9% |
| Riboflavin | 0.066 mg | 5% |
| Thiamin | 0..072 mg | 6% |

| Minerals | Value | RDA% |
|---|---|---|
| Calcium | 44 mg | 4% |
| Copper | 0.231 mg | 27% |
| Iron | 1.28 mg | 16% |
| Magnesium | 60 mg | 15% |
| Manganese | 0.256 mg | 11% |
| Phosphorus | 90 mg | 13% |
| Selenium | 0.3 µg | <0.5% |
| Zinc | 0.49 mg | 8% |

# *Arugula*

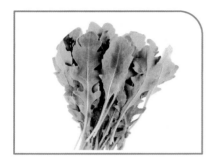

## How to store?

Loosely wrap Arugula in damp paper towels and place in a plastic bag for up to 3 days in the fridge.

## Benefits:

- Protect the eyes
- Improve digestion
- Inprove bone health
- Improve babies brain health

## NUTRITIONAL RATIO

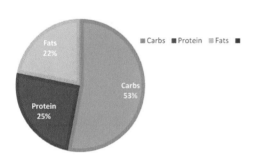

■ Carbs ■ Protein ■ Fats ■

Fats 22%

Carbs 53%

Protein 25%

### Nutrition Values for 100g

**Energy:** 25 Kcal

**Carbohydrate:** 3.65 g

**Protein:** 2.58 g

**Total fat:** 0.66 g

**Dietary fiber:** 1.6 g

| Vitamin | Value | RDA % |
|---|---|---|
| Vitamin A | 2373 IU | 79% |
| Vitamin C | 15 mg | 25% |
| Vitamin E | 0.43 mg | 3% |
| Vitamin K | 108.6 µg | 90% |
| Folates | 97 µg | 24% |
| Niancin | 0.305 mg | 2% |
| Pantothenic acid | 0.437 mg | 8% |
| Pyridoxine | 0.073 mg | 6% |
| Riboflavin | 0.086 mg | 7% |
| Thiamin | 0.044 mg | 4% |

| Minerals | Value | RDA% |
|---|---|---|
| Calcium | 160 mg | 16% |
| Copper | 0.076 mg | 8% |
| Iron | 1.46 mg | 18% |
| Magnesium | 47 mg | 12% |
| Manganese | 0.321 mg | 14% |
| Phosphorus | 52 mg | 7.5% |
| Selenium | 0.3 µg | <1% |
| Zinc | 0.47 mg | 8% |

# *Asparagus*

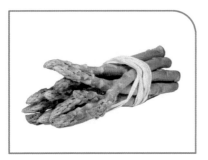

## How to store?

Stand spears in 2.5 cm (1") of water or wrap ends with damp paper towel. Cover, refrigerate for up to four days.

## Benefits:

- Antioxydant agent
- Improve fertility
- Inprove digestion
- Good for the skin
- Help lower blood pressure

## NUTRITIONAL RATIO

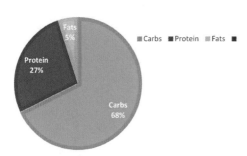

Carbs ■ Protein ■ Fats ■

### Nutrition Values for 100g

**Energy:** 20 Kcal

**Carbohydrate:** 3.38 g

**Protein:** 2.20 g

**Total fat:** 0.12 g

**Dietary fiber:** 2.1 g

| Vitamin | Value | RDA % |
|---|---|---|
| Vitamin A | 756 IU | 25% |
| Vitamin C | 5.6 mg | 9% |
| Vitamin E | 1.13 mg | 7.5% |
| Vitamin K | 41.6 µg | 35% |
| Folates | 52 µg | 13% |
| Niancin | 0.978 mg | 6% |
| Pantothenic acid | 0.274 mg | 5% |
| Pyridoxine | 0.091 mg | 7% |
| Riboflavin | 0.141 mg | 11% |
| Thiamin | 0.143 mg | 12% |

| Minerals | Value | RDA% |
|---|---|---|
| Calcium | 24 mg | 2.5% |
| Copper | 0.189 mg | 21% |
| Iron | 1.14 mg | 14% |
| Magnesium | 14 mg | 1% |
| Manganese | 0.158 mg | 7% |
| Phosphorus | 52 mg | 7.5% |
| Selenium | 2.3 µg | 4% |
| Zinc | 0.54 mg | 5% |

# *Bamboo Shoots*

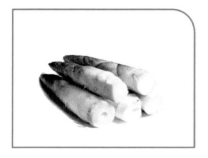

### How to store?

Fresh bamboo shoots can be stored in plastic bags in the refrigerator for up to 2 weeks. They can also be cooked then frozen.

### Benefits:

- Balance Cholesterol Levels
- Wound cleaner
- Anti-inflammatory Properties
- Protect the heart
- Anti-venomous (Snake & Scorpion)

## NUTRITIONAL RATIO

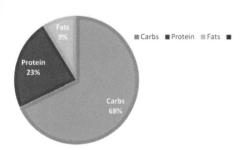

■ Carbs  ■ Protein  ■ Fats  ■

### Nutrition Values for 100g

**Energy:** 27 Kcal

**Carbohydrate:** 5.2 g

**Protein:** 2.60 g

**Total fat:** 0.3 g

**Dietary fiber:** 2.2 g

| Vitamin | Value | RDA % |
|---|---|---|
| Vitamin A | 20 IU | <1% |
| Vitamin C | 4 mg | 7% |
| Vitamin E | 1mg | 7% |
| Folates | 7 µg | 2% |
| Niancin | 0.600 mg | 4% |
| Pantothenic acid | 0.161 mg | 3% |
| Pyridoxine | 0.240 mg | 18% |
| Riboflavin | 0.070 mg | 5% |
| Thiamin | 0.150 mg | 12% |

| Minerals | Value | RDA% |
|---|---|---|
| Calcium | 13 mg | 1.5% |
| Copper | 0.190 mg | 21% |
| Iron | 0.50 mg | 6% |
| Magnesium | 3 mg | <1% |
| Manganese | 0.262 mg | 11% |
| Phosphorus | 59 mg | 8% |
| Selenium | 0.8 µg | 1.5 % |
| Zinc | 1.10 mg | 10% |

# *Beans (Green)*

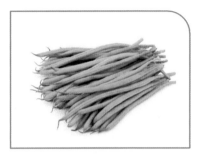

### How to store?

Cover, refrigerate unwashed for up to five days.

### Benefits:

- Reduce heart diseases
- Control diabetes
- Boost immunity
- Prevent colon cancer
- Eye Care

## NUTRITIONAL RATIO

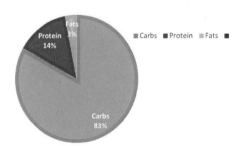

Carbs  Protein  Fats

Fats 3%
Protein 14%
Carbs 83%

## Nutrition Values for 100g

**Energy:** 31 Kcal

**Carbohydrate:** 7.13 g

**Protein:** 1.82 g

**Total fat:** 0.34 g

**Dietary fiber:** 3.4 g

| Vitamin | Value | RDA % |
|---|---|---|
| Vitamin A | 690 IU | 23% |
| Vitamin C | 16.3 mg | 27% |
| Vitamin K | 14.4 µg | 12% |
| Folates | 37 µg | 9% |
| Niacin | 0.752 mg | 5% |
| Pantothenic acid | 0.094 mg | 2% |
| Pyridoxine | 0.074 mg | 5.5% |
| Riboflavin | 0.105 mg | 8% |
| Thiamin | 0..084 mg | 7% |

| Minerals | Value | RDA% |
|---|---|---|
| Calcium | 37 mg | 3.7% |
| Iron | 1.04 mg | 13% |
| Magnesium | 25 mg | 6% |
| Manganese | 0.214 mg | 9% |
| Phosphorus | 38 mg | 6% |
| Zinc | 0.24 mg | 2% |

# *Beets*

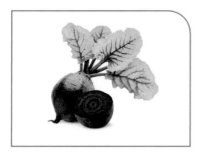

### How to store?

Refrigerate unwashed with stem and root attached, covered for up to 1 week.

### Benefits:

- Anti-Aging
- Low the blood pressure
- Inprove digestion
- Reduce birth defect
- Improve liver detoxification

## NUTRITIONAL RATIO

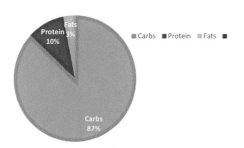

■ Carbs  ■ Protein  ■ Fats  ■

Protein 10%
Fats 3%
Carbs 87%

### Nutrition Values for 100g

**Energy:** 43 Kcal

**Carbohydrate:** 9.56 g

**Protein:** 1.61 g

**Total fat:** 0.17 g

**Dietary fiber:** 2.80 g

| Vitamin | Value | RDA % |
|---|---|---|
| Vitamin A | 33 IU | 1% |
| Vitamin C | 4.9 mg | 8% |
| Vitamin E | 0.04 mg | 0.5% |
| Vitamin K | 0.2 µg | 0% |
| Folates | 109 µg | 27% |
| Niacin | 0.334 mg | 2% |
| Pantothenic acid | 0.155 mg | 3% |
| Pyridoxine | 0.067 mg | 5% |
| Riboflavin | 0.057 mg | 4% |
| Thiamin | 0.031 mg | 2.5% |

| Minerals | Value | RDA% |
|---|---|---|
| Calcium | 16 mg | 1.5% |
| Copper | 0.075 mg | 8% |
| Iron | 0.80 mg | 10% |
| Magnesium | 23 mg | 6% |
| Manganese | 0.329 mg | 14% |
| Zinc | 0.35 mg | 3% |

# *Belgian Endive*

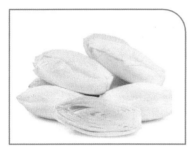

## How to store?

Store Belgian endives wrapped in a damp paper towel inside a plastic bag in the refrigerator for three to five days. Do not wash until ready to use.

## Benefits:

- Improve brain health
- Manage cholestrol levels
- Improve vision
- Promote strong bones
- help with diabetes

## NUTRITIONAL RATIO

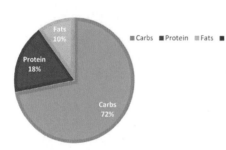

Carbs ■ Protein ■ Fats ■

### Nutrition Values for 100g

**Energy:** 17 Kcal

**Carbohydrate:** 3.35 g

**Protein:** 1.25 g

**Total fat:** 0.20 g

**Dietary fiber:** 3.10 g

| Vitamin | Value | RDA % |
|---|---|---|
| Vitamin A | 2167 IU | 72% |
| Vitamin C | 6.5 mg | 11% |
| Vitamin E | 0.44 mg | 3% |
| Vitamin K | 231 µg | 192% |
| Folates | 142 µg | 36% |
| Niancin | 0.400 mg | 2.5% |
| Pantothenic acid | 0.900 mg | 18% |
| Pyridoxine | 0.020 mg | 1.5% |
| Riboflavin | 0.075 mg | 6% |
| Thiamin | 0..080 mg | 7% |

| Minerals | Value | RDA% |
|---|---|---|
| Calcium | 52 mg | 5% |
| Copper | 0.099 mg | 11% |
| Iron | 0.83 mg | 10% |
| Magnesium | 15 mg | 4% |
| Manganese | 0.420 mg | 18% |
| Phosphorus | 28 mg | 4% |
| Selenium | 0.2 µg | 1% |
| Zinc | 0.79 mg | 7% |

# *Bitter Melon*

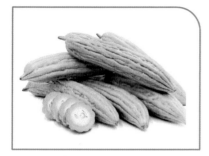

## How to store?

Store melon loose in a paper or plastic bag in the refrigerator for 3 to 5 days. Slice the melon only immediately before use.

## Benefits:

- Blood purification
- Hemorrhoid Relief
- Antifungal Agent
- Improve immunity
- Asthma Relief

## NUTRITIONAL RATIO

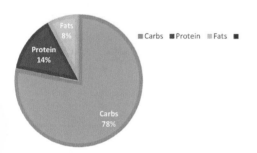

■ Carbs  ■ Protein  ■ Fats  ■

Fats 8%
Protein 14%
Carbs 78%

## Nutrition Values for 100g

**Energy:** 17 Kcal

**Carbohydrate:** 3.70 g

**Protein:** 1.00 g

**Total fat:** 0.17 g

**Dietary fiber:** 2.80 g

| Vitamin | Value | RDA % |
|---|---|---|
| Vitamin A | 471 IU | 16% |
| Vitamin C | 84 mg | 140% |
| Folates | 72 µg | 18% |
| Niacin | 0.400 mg | 2.5% |
| Pantothenic acid | 0.212 mg | 4% |
| Pyridoxine | 0.043 mg | 15% |
| Riboflavin | 0.040 mg | 12% |
| Thiamin | 0..040 mg | 2% |

| Minerals | Value | RDA% |
|---|---|---|
| Calcium | 19 mg | 2% |
| Copper | 0.034 mg | 4% |
| Iron | 0.43 mg | 5% |
| Magnesium | 17 mg | 4% |
| Manganese | 0.089 mg | 4% |
| Zinc | 0.80 mg | 7% |

# *Bok Choy*

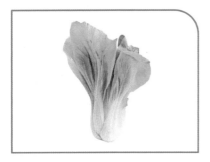

## How to store?

Store bok choy in a plastic bag in the crisper section of your refrigerator for up to a week. Wash immediately before using.

## Benefits:

- Improves Bone Strength
- Eye Care
- Prevents Chronic Disease
- Skin Care
- Improves Cardiovascular Health

## NUTRITIONAL RATIO

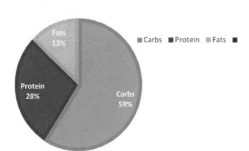

Carbs 59%
Protein 28%
Fats 13%

### Nutrition Values for 100g

**Energy:** 13 Kcal

**Carbohydrate:** 2.18 g

**Protein:** 1.5 g

**Total fat:** 0.20 g

**Dietary fiber:** 1 g

| Vitamin | Value | RDA % |
|---|---|---|
| Vitamin A | 4468 IU | 149% |
| Vitamin C | 45 mg | 75% |
| Vitamin K | 45.5 µg | 38% |
| Folates | 66 µg | 16% |
| Niancin | 0.500 mg | 3% |
| Pantothenic acid | 0.088 mg | 1.5% |
| Pyridoxine | 0.194 mg | 15% |
| Riboflavin | 0.070 mg | 5% |
| Thiamin | 0..040 mg | 3.5% |

| Minerals | Value | RDA% |
|---|---|---|
| Calcium | 105 mg | 10.5% |
| Copper | 0.80 mg | 10% |
| Magnesium | 19 mg | 5% |
| Manganese | 0.159 mg | 7% |
| Phosphorus | 37 mg | 5% |
| Zinc | 0.19 mg | 1.5% |

# *Broadbeans*

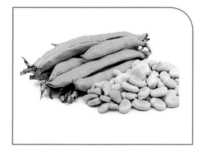

## How to store?

Place them in a plastic bag in the crisper section of the refrigerator right away. The pods will keep for five to seven days in the refrigerator.

## Benefits:

• Prevent Osteoporosis     • Prevent birth defects

• Boost Immunity     • Boost Immunity

• Promote hearth health

## NUTRITIONAL RATIO

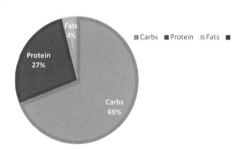

■ Carbs ■ Protein ■ Fats ■

### Nutrition Values for 100g

**Energy:** 341 Kcal

**Carbohydrate:** 58.59 g

**Protein:** 26.12 g

**Total fat:** 1.53 g

**Dietary fiber:** 25 g

| Vitamin | Value | RDA % |
|---|---|---|
| Vitamin A | 53 IU | 2% |
| Vitamin C | 1.4 mg | 2% |
| Vitamin K | 9 µg | 7.5% |
| Folates | 423 µg | 106% |
| Niancin | 2.832 mg | 18% |
| Pantothenic acid | 0.976 mg | 19.5% |
| Pyridoxine | 0.366 mg | 28% |
| Riboflavin | 0.333 mg | 25% |
| Thiamin | 0.555 mg | 46.25% |

| Minerals | Value | RDA% |
|---|---|---|
| Calcium | 103 mg | 10% |
| Copper | 0.824 mg | 42% |
| Iron | 6.70 mg | 84% |
| Magnesium | 192 mg | 18% |
| Manganese | 1.626 mg | 71% |
| Phosphorus | 421 mg | 60% |
| Selenium | 8.2 µg | 15% |
| Zinc | 3.14 mg | 9% |

# *Broccoli*

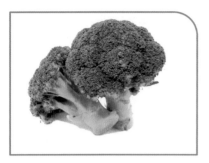

## How to store?

Cover, refrigerate unwashed for up to five days.

## Benefits:

- Aids in digestion
- Controls diabetes
- Anti-inflammatory properties
- Reduce allergies
- Detoxifies the body

## NUTRITIONAL RATIO

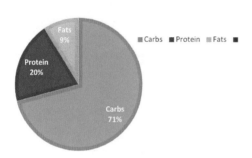

Carbs | Protein | Fats

Fats 9%
Protein 20%
Carbs 71%

### Nutrition Values for 100g

**Energy:** 34 Kcal

**Carbohydrate:** 6.64 g

**Protein:** 2.82 g

**Total fat:** 0.37 g

**Dietary fiber:** 2.60 g

| Vitamin | Value | RDA % |
|---------|-------|-------|
| Vitamin A | 623 IU | 21% |
| Vitamin C | 89.2 mg | 149% |
| Vitamin E | 0.17 mg | 1.5% |
| Vitamin K | 101.6 µg | 85% |
| Folates | 63 µg | 16% |
| Niancin | 0.639 mg | 4% |
| Pantothenic acid | 0.573 mg | 12% |
| Pyridoxine | 0.175 mg | 13% |
| Riboflavin | 0.117 mg | 9% |
| Thiamin | 0..071 mg | 6% |

| Minerals | Value | RDA% |
|----------|-------|------|
| Calcium | 47 mg | 5% |
| Copper | 0.049 mg | 5.5% |
| Iron | 0.73 mg | 9% |
| Magnesium | 21 mg | 5% |
| Manganese | 0.210 mg | 9% |
| Selenium | 2.5 µg | 5% |
| Zinc | 0.41 mg | 4% |

# *Broccoli Rabe*

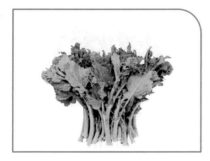

### How to store?

Store in a bag in the refrigerator for up to one week.

### Benefits:

- Controls diabetes
- Protects the heart
- Prevents cancer
- Lowers Neural Tube Defects
- Improve bone strength

## NUTRITIONAL RATIO

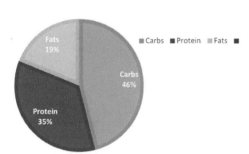

■ Carbs ■ Protein ■ Fats ■

### Nutrition Values for 100g

**Energy:** 22 Kcal

**Carbohydrate:** 2.85 g

**Protein:** 3.17 g

**Total fat:** 0.49 g

**Dietary fiber:** 2.7 g

| Vitamin | Value | RDA % |
|---|---|---|
| Vitamin A | 2622 IU | 87% |
| Vitamin C | 20.2 mg | 34% |
| Vitamine E | 1.62 mg | 11% |
| Vitamin K | 224 µg | 186% |
| Folates | 83 µg | 21% |
| Niancin | 1.221 mg | 5% |
| Pantothenic acid | 0.210 mg | 7.5% |
| Pyridoxine | 0.171 mg | 14% |
| Riboflavin | 0.129 mg | 10% |
| Thiamin | 0.162 mg | 13.5% |

| Minerals | Value | RDA% |
|---|---|---|
| Calcium | 108 mg | 11% |
| Copper | 0.042 mg | 5% |
| Iron | 2.14 mg | 27% |
| Magnesium | 22 mg | 5% |
| Manganese | 0.395 mg | 17% |
| Selenium | 1 µg | 1.5% |
| Zinc | 0.77 mg | 7% |

# *Brussel Sprouts*

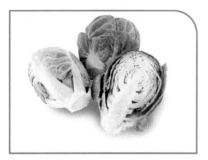

### How to store?

Cover, refrigerate unwashed for up to five days.

### Benefits:

- Boosts Immune System
- Helps in Blood Clotting
- Inprove digestion
- Lowers Inflammation
- Increases your Metabolism

## NUTRITIONAL RATIO

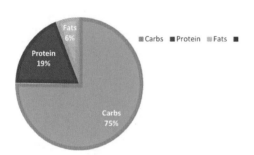

Carbs  Protein  Fats

### Nutrition Values for 100g

**Energy:** 43 Kcal

**Carbohydrate:** 8.95 g

**Protein:** 3.38 g

**Total fat:** 0.30 g

**Dietary fiber:** 3.80 g

| Vitamin | Value | RDA % |
|---|---|---|
| Vitamin A | 754 IU | 25% |
| Vitamin C | 85 mg | 142% |
| Vitamin K | 177 µg | 147% |
| Folates | 61 µg | 15% |
| Niancin | 0.745 mg | 4.5% |
| Pantothenic acid | 0.309 mg | 6% |
| Pyridoxine | 0.219 mg | 17% |
| Riboflavin | 0.90 mg | 7% |
| Thiamin | 0.139 mg | 13% |

| Minerals | Value | RDA% |
|---|---|---|
| Calcium | 42 mg | 4% |
| Copper | 0.70 mg | 8% |
| Iron | 1.40 mg | 17.5% |
| Magnesium | 23 mg | 6% |
| Manganese | 0.337 mg | 15% |
| Phosphorus | 69 mg | 10% |
| Selenium | 1.6 µg | 3% |
| Zinc | 0.42 mg | 4% |

# *Cabbage ( Green)*

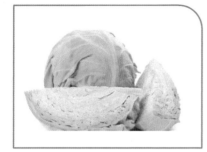

**How to store?**

Cover, refrigerate unwashed for up to two weeks.

**Benefits:**

- Antioxydant agent
- Anti-inflammatory Agent
- Regulates Cholesterol
- Hair & skin care
- Protects from Radiation Therapy

## NUTRITIONAL RATIO

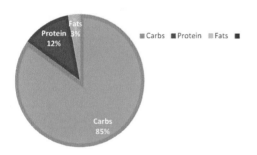

■ Carbs  ■ Protein  ■ Fats  ■

### Nutrition Values for 100g

**Energy:** 25 Kcal

**Carbohydrate:** 5.8 g

**Protein:** 1.3 g

**Total fat:** 0.1 g

**Dietary fiber:** 2.50 g

| Vitamin | Value | RDA % |
|---|---|---|
| Vitamin A | 98 IU | 3% |
| Vitamin C | 36.6 mg | 61% |
| Vitamin K | 76 µg | 63% |
| Folates | 53 µg | 13% |
| Niancin | 0.234 mg | 1.5% |
| Pantothenic acid | 0.212 mg | 4% |
| Pyridoxine | 0.124 mg | 10% |
| Riboflavin | 0.040 mg | 3% |
| Thiamin | 0.061 mg | 5% |

| Minerals | Value | RDA% |
|---|---|---|
| Calcium | 40 mg | 4% |
| Iron | 0.47 mg | 6% |
| Magnesium | 12 mg | 3% |
| Manganese | 0.160 mg | 7% |
| Phosphorus | 26mg | 3.5% |
| Zinc | 0.18 mg | 1.5% |

# *Cabbage (Red)*

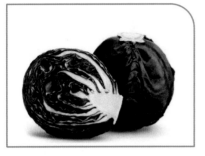

### How to store?

Cover, refrigerate unwashed for up to one week.

### Benefits:

- Anti-aging property
- Treats uclers
- Boosts Immune System
- Protects from Alzheimer
- Increases Bone Mineral Density

## NUTRITIONAL RATIO

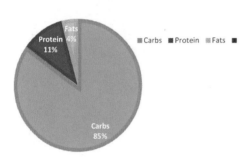

■ Carbs ■ Protein ■ Fats ■

### Nutrition Values for 100g

**Energy:** 31 Kcal

**Carbohydrate:** 26.2 g

**Protein:** 1.4 g

**Total fat:** 0.2 g

**Dietary fiber:** 2.1 g

| Vitamin | Value | RDA % |
|---|---|---|
| Vitamin A | 1116 IU | 22% |
| Vitamin C | 57 mg | 95% |
| Vitamin E | 0.1 mg | 1% |
| Vitamin K | 38.2 µg | 48% |
| Folates | 18 µg | 5% |
| Niancin | 0.4 mg | 2% |
| Pantothenic acid | 0.1 mg | 1% |
| Riboflavin | 0.1 mg | 4% |
| Thiamin | 0.1 mg | 4% |

| Minerals | Value | RDA% |
|---|---|---|
| Calcium | 45 mg | 4% |
| Iron | 0.8 mg | 4% |
| Magnesium | 16 mg | 4% |
| Manganese | 0.2 mg | 12% |
| Phosphorus | 30 mg | 3% |
| Selenium | 0.6 µg | 1% |
| Zinc | 0.2 mg | 1% |

# *Carrots*

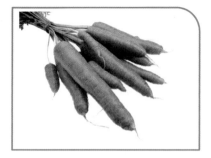

## How to store?

Remove green leafy tops. Cover, refrigerate unwashed young carrots for up to two weeks. Mature carrots keep 3 to 4 weeks.

## Benefits:

- Regulate Blood Cholesterol
- Improve Eye Health
- Control Diabetes
- Lower Blood Pressure
- Improve Oral Health

## NUTRITIONAL RATIO

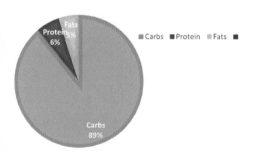

■ Carbs ■ Protein ■ Fats ■

### Nutrition Values for 100g

**Energy:** 41 Kcal

**Carbohydrate:** 9.58 g

**Protein:** 0.93 g

**Total fat:** 0.24 g

**Dietary fiber:** 2.8 g

| Vitamin | Value | RDA % |
|---|---|---|
| Vitamin A | 16706 IU | 577% |
| Vitamin C | 5.9 mg | 10% |
| Vitamin K | 13.2 µg | 11% |
| Folates | 19 µg | 5% |
| Niancin | 0.983 mg | 6% |
| Pantothenic acid | 0.273 mg | 5.5% |
| Pyridoxine | 0.138 mg | 10% |
| Riboflavin | 0.058 mg | 4% |
| Thiamin | 0.066 mg | 6% |

| Minerals | Value | RDA% |
|---|---|---|
| Calcium | 33 mg | 3% |
| Copper | 0.045 mg | 5% |
| Iron | 0.30 mg | 4% |
| Magnesium | 12 mg | 3% |
| Manganese | 0.143 mg | 6% |
| Phosphorus | 35 mg | 5% |
| Selenium | 0.1 µg | 1% |
| Zinc | 0.24 mg | 2% |

# Cassava (Yuca Root)

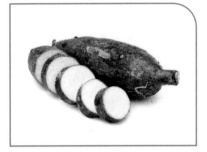

### How to store?

Store unpeeled in a cool, dark, dry place for up to 1 week. Peeled yucca root can be stored in water in the refrigerator – it will last for 1 month if you change the water every two days- or wrapped tightly and frozen for several months.

### Benefits:

- Antioxydant agent
- Controls Diabetes

## NUTRITIONAL RATIO

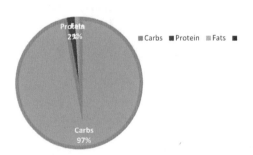

Protein 2%
Carbs 97%

■ Carbs ■ Protein ■ Fats ■

### Nutrition Values for 100g

**Energy:** 160 Kcal

**Carbohydrate:** 38.06 g

**Protein:** 1.36 g

**Total fat:** 0.28 g

**Dietary fiber:** 1.8 g

| Vitamin | Value | RDA % |
|---------|-------|-------|
| Vitamin A | 13 IU | 1% |
| Vitamin C | 20.6 mg | 34% |
| Vitamin E | 0.19 | 1% |
| Vitamin K | 1.9 µg | 1.5% |
| Folates | 27 µg | 7% |
| Niancin | 0.854 mg | 5% |
| Pyridoxine | 0.088 mg | 7% |
| Riboflavin | 0.048 mg | 4% |
| Thiamin | 0..087 mg | 7% |

| Minerals | Value | RDA% |
|----------|-------|------|
| Calcium | 16 mg | 1.6% |
| Iron | 0.27 mg | 3% |
| Magnesium | 21 mg | 5% |
| Manganese | 0.383 mg | 1.5% |
| Phosphorus | 27 mg | 4% |
| Zinc | 0.34 mg | 3% |

# *Cauliflower*

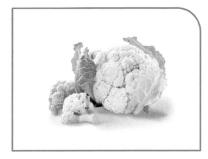

**How to store?**

Cover, refrigerate unwashed for up to one week.

**Benefits:**

• Prevents Oxidative Stress   • Iron Absorption

• Improves Bone Health   • Detoxifies the Body

• Improves Cardiovascular Health

## NUTRITIONAL RATIO

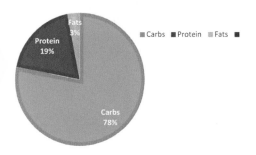

■ Carbs ■ Protein ■ Fats ■

Fats 3%
Protein 19%
Carbs 78%

### Nutrition Values for 100g

**Energy:** 25 Kcal

**Carbohydrate:** 4.97 g

**Protein:** 1.92 g

**Total fat:** 0.28 g

**Dietary fiber:** 2.0 g

| Vitamin | Value | RDA % |
|---|---|---|
| Vitamin C | 48.2 mg | 80% |
| Vitamin E | 0.08 mg | 0.5% |
| Vitamin K | 15.5 µg | 13% |
| Folates | 57 µg | 14% |
| Niancin | 0.507 mg | 3% |
| Pantothenic acid | 0.667 mg | 13% |
| Pyridoxine | 0.184 mg | 14% |
| Riboflavin | 0.060 mg | 4.5% |
| Thiamin | 0..050 mg | 4% |

| Minerals | Value | RDA% |
|---|---|---|
| Calcium | 22 mg | 2% |
| Copper | 0.039 mg | 4.5% |
| Iron | 0.42 mg | 5% |
| Magnesium | 15 mg | 3.5% |
| Manganese | 0.155 mg | 7% |
| Zinc | 0.27 mg | 2.5% |

# *Celeriac*

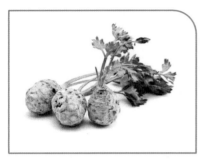

### How to store?

Trim off stalks and refrigerate unwashed, covered for up to a week.

### Benefits:

• Lowers Cholesterol Level    • Reduces Blood Pressure

• Reduces Asthma Symptoms    • Lowers Arthritis Pain

• Prevents Urinary Tract Infections

## NUTRITIONAL RATIO

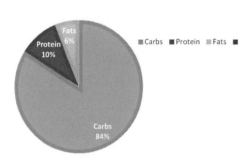

Carbs   Protein   Fats

### Nutrition Values for 100g

**Energy:** 42 Kcal

**Carbohydrate:** 9.20 g

**Protein:** 1.5 g

**Total fat:** 0.30 g

**Dietary fiber:** 1.8 g

| Vitamin | Value | RDA % |
|---|---|---|
| Vitamin C | 8 mg | 13% |
| Vitamin E | 0.36 mg | 2% |
| Vitamin K | 41 µg | 34% |
| Folates | 8 µg | 2% |
| Niancin | 0.700 mg | 4% |
| Pantothenic acid | 0.352 mg | 6% |
| Pyridoxine | 0.165 mg | 13% |
| Riboflavin | 0.060 mg | 5% |
| Thiamin | 0..050 mg | 4% |

| Minerals | Value | RDA% |
|---|---|---|
| Calcium | 43 mg | 4.3% |
| Copper | 0.070 mg | 8% |
| Iron | 0.70 mg | 9% |
| Magnesium | 20 mg | 5% |
| Manganese | 0.158 mg | 7% |
| Phosphorus | 115 mg | 16% |
| Zinc | 0.33 mg | 3% |

*Celery*

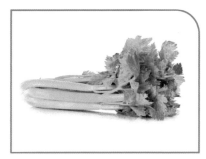

### How to store?

Cover, refrigerate unwashed for up to two weeks.

### Benefits:

- Lowers inflammation
- Prevents liver diseases
- Treats high blood pressure
- Prevent uclers
- Fights infections

## NUTRITIONAL RATIO

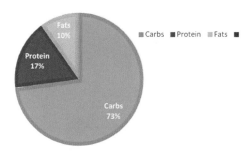

■ Carbs  ■ Protein  ■ Fats  ■

### Nutrition Values for 100g

**Energy:** 16 Kcal

**Carbohydrate:** 3 g

**Protein:** 3.46 g

**Total fat:** 1.12 g

**Dietary fiber:** 2.10 g

| Vitamin | Value | RDA % |
|---|---|---|
| Vitamin A | 449IU | 15% |
| Vitamin C | 3.1 mg | 5% |
| Vitamin K | 29.3 µg | 24% |
| Folates | 36 µg | 9% |
| Niacin | 0.320 mg | 2% |
| Pantothenic acid | 0.246 mg | 5% |
| Pyridoxine | 0.074 mg | 6% |
| Riboflavin | 0.57 mg | 4% |
| Thiamin | 0..021 mg | 2% |

| Minerals | Value | RDA% |
|---|---|---|
| Calcium | 40 mg | 4% |
| Copper | 0.35 mg | 4% |
| Iron | 0.20 mg | 2.5% |
| Magnesium | 11 mg | 3% |
| Manganese | 0.103 mg | 4.5% |
| Phosphorus | 24 mg | 3% |
| Zinc | 0.13 mg | 1% |

# *Chayote*

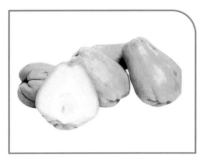

### How to store?

Refrigerate unwashed, covered for up to one week.

### Benefits:

- Lower cholesterol
- Prevents anemia
- Prevents constipation
- Prevents heart diseases
- Prevents premature aging

## NUTRITIONAL RATIO

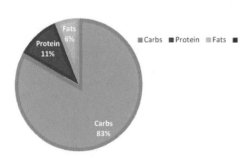

Carbs ■ Protein ■ Fats ■

Fats 6%
Protein 11%
Carbs 83%

### Nutrition Values for 100g

**Energy:** 19 Kcal

**Carbohydrate:** 4.51 g

**Protein:** 0.82g

**Total fat:** 0.13 g

**Dietary fiber:** 1.7 g

| Vitamin | Value | RDA % |
|---|---|---|
| Vitamin C | 7.7 mg | 13% |
| Vitamin E | 0.12 mg | <1% |
| Vitamin K | 4.1 µg | 4% |
| Folates | 93 µg | 23% |
| Niancin | 0.470 mg | 3% |
| Pantothenic acid | 0.249 mg | 5% |
| Pyridoxine | 0.076 mg | 6% |
| Riboflavin | 0.029 mg | 2% |
| Thiamin | 0..025 mg | 2% |

| Minerals | Value | RDA% |
|---|---|---|
| Calcium | 17 mg | 1.7% |
| Iron | 0.34 mg | 4% |
| Magnesium | 12 mg | 3% |
| Manganese | 0.189 mg | 8% |
| Phosphorus | 18 mg | 2.5% |
| Selenium | 0.2 µg | <1% |
| Zinc | 0.74 mg | 7% |

*Chicory*

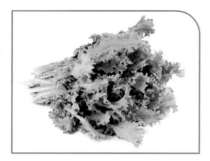

**How to store?**

They are more enjoyable when combined with other vegetables. Its strong taste enhances spring mixes or salads of greens and can also be used to garnish cheese platters or smoked fish. Eat it braised, raw, sautéed or stewed.

**Benefits:**

- Aids in Digestion
- Reduces Arthritis Pain

## NUTRITIONAL RATIO

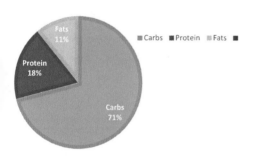

Carbs ▪ Protein ▪ Fats ▪

- Fats 11%
- Protein 18%
- Carbs 71%

### Nutrition Values for 100g

**Energy:** 23 Kcal

**Carbohydrate:** 4.70 g

**Protein:** 1.7 g

**Total fat:** 0.30 g

**Dietary fiber:** 4 g

| Vitamin | Value | RDA % |
|---------|-------|-------|
| Vitamin A | 5.717 IU | 190% |
| Vitamin C | 24 mg | 40% |
| Vitamin E | 2.26 mg | 15% |
| Vitamin K | 297 µg | 215% |
| Folates | 110 µg | 27% |
| Niacin | 0.500 mg | 3% |
| Pyridoxine | 0.105 mg | 8% |
| Riboflavin | 0.100 mg | 7.7% |
| Thiamin | 0..060 mg | 5% |

| Minerals | Value | RDA% |
|----------|-------|------|
| Calcium | 100 mg | 10% |
| Copper | 0.295 mg | 33% |
| Iron | 0.90 mg | 11% |
| Magnesium | 30 mg | 8% |
| Manganese | 0.429 mg | 18% |
| Phosphorus | 45 mg | 9% |

# *Collards*

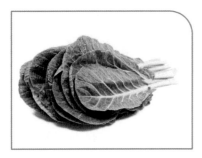

### How to store?

Refrigerate collard greens in a plastic bag for up to 5 days.

### Benefits:

- Improve dgestion
- Improve sleep & mood
- Inprove bone health
- Improve immune system
- promote healthy looking skin and hair

## NUTRITIONAL RATIO

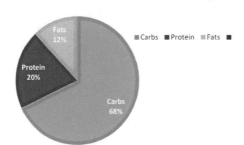

Carbs — Protein — Fats

- Fats 12%
- Protein 20%
- Carbs 68%

### Nutrition Values for 100g

**Energy:** 32 Kcal

**Carbohydrate:** 5.42 g

**Protein:** 3.02 g

**Total fat:** 0.61 g

**Dietary fiber:** 4 g

| Vitamin | Value | RDA % |
|---|---|---|
| Vitamin A | 5019 IU | 170% |
| Vitamin C | 35.3 mg | 59% |
| Vitamin E | 2.26 mg | 15% |
| Vitamin K | 437.1 µg | 37% |
| Folates | 129 µg | 32% |
| Niancin | 0.742 mg | 5% |
| Pantothenic acid | 0.267 mg | 5% |
| Pyridoxine | 0.165 mg | 13% |
| Riboflavin | 0.130 mg | 10% |
| Thiamin | 0.054 mg | 4.5% |

| Minerals | Value | RDA% |
|---|---|---|
| Calcium | 232 mg | 23% |
| Copper | 0.039 mg | 4.5% |
| Iron | 0.47 mg | 6% |
| Magnesium | 27 mg | 7% |
| Manganese | 0.658 mg | 30% |
| Phosphorus | 1.3 µg | 2% |
| Zinc | 0.21 mg | 2% |

# *Corn*

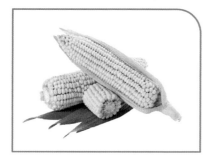

## How to store?

Wrap unhusked ears with damp paper towel. Cover, refrigerate for up to two days.

## Benefits:

- Prevents Hemorrhoids
- Protects Your Heart
- Lowers LDL Cholesterol
- Prevents Anemia
- Eye & Skin Care
- Controls Diabetes

## NUTRITIONAL RATIO

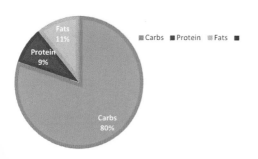

Carbs • Protein • Fats •

Fats 11%
Protein 9%
Carbs 80%

### Nutrition Values for 100g

**Energy:** 86 Kcal

**Carbohydrate:** 18.70 g

**Protein:** 3.27 g

**Total fat:** 1.35 g

**Dietary fiber:** 2.0 g

| Vitamin | Value | RDA % |
|---|---|---|
| Vitamin A | 187 IU | 6% |
| Vitamin C | 6.8 mg | 11% |
| Vitamin E | 0.07 mg | <1% |
| Vitamin K | 0.3 µg | 2% |
| Folates | 42 µg | 10.5% |
| Niacin | 1.770 mg | 11% |
| Pantothenic acid | 0.717 mg | 14% |
| Pyridoxine | 0.093 mg | 7% |
| Riboflavin | 0.055 mg | 4% |
| Thiamin | 0.155 mg | 13% |

| Minerals | Value | RDA% |
|---|---|---|
| Calcium | 2 mg | <1% |
| Copper | 0.054 mg | 6% |
| Iron | 0.52 mg | 6.5% |
| Magnesium | 37 mg | 9% |
| Manganese | 0.163 mg | 7% |
| Selenium | 0.6 µg | 1% |
| Zinc | 0.46 mg | 4% |

# *Crookneck*

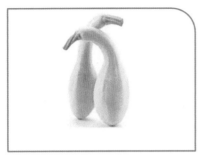

## How to store?

Store unwashed in a plastic bag in the refrigerator for up to a week.

## Benefits:

- Treats Asthma
- Prevents Infections
- Improve vision
- Manages Diabetes
- Protects Heart Health

### NUTRITIONAL RATIO

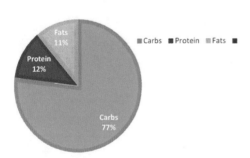

Carbs  Protein  Fats

Fats 11%
Protein 12%
Carbs 77%

### Nutrition Values for 100g

**Energy:** 14 Kcal

**Carbohydrate:** 4.0 g

**Protein:** 0.9 g

**Total fat:** 0.2 g

**Dietary fiber:** 1.9 g

| Vitamin | Value | RDA % |
|---|---|---|
| Vitamin A | 150 IU | 3% |
| Vitamin C | 8.4 mg | 14% |
| Folates | 23 µg | 6% |
| Niancin | 0.5 mg | 2% |
| Pantothenic acid | 0.1 mg | 1% |
| Pyridoxine | 0.192 mg | 15% |
| Thiamin | 0.1 mg | 3% |

| Minerals | Value | RDA% |
|---|---|---|
| Calcium | 21 mg | 2% |
| Copper | 0.1 mg | 5% |
| Iron | 0.5 mg | 3% |
| Magnesium | 21 mg | 5% |
| Manganese | 0.2 mg | 8% |
| Phosphorus | 32 mg | 3% |
| Selenium | 0.2 µg | 0% |
| Zinc | 0.3 mg | 2% |

# *Cucumber*

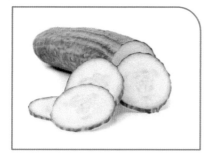

**How to store?**

Refrigerate unwashed for up to one week.

**Benefits:**

- Manage Diabetes
- Control Blood Pressure
- Prevents  Kidney Stones
- prevents inflammation
- Prevents constipation

## NUTRITIONAL RATIO

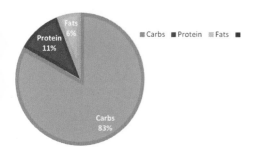

■ Carbs  ■ Protein  ■ Fats  ■

### Nutrition Values for 100g

**Energy:** 15 Kcal

**Carbohydrate:** 3.63 g

**Protein:** 0.65 g

**Total fat:** 0.11 g

**Dietary fiber:** 0.5 g

| Vitamin | Value | RDA % |
|---|---|---|
| Vitamin A | 105 IU | 3.5% |
| Vitamin C | 2.8 mg | 4.5% |
| Vitamin E | 0.03 mg | 0% |
| Vitamin K | 16.4 µg | 13.6% |
| Folates | 7 µg | 2% |
| Niacin | 0.098 mg | <1% |
| Pantothenic acid | 0.259 mg | 5% |
| Pyridoxine | 0.040 mg | 3% |
| Riboflavin | 0.033 mg | 3% |
| Thiamin | 0..027 mg | 2% |

| Minerals | Value | RDA% |
|---|---|---|
| Calcium | 16 mg | 1.6% |
| Iron | 0.28 mg | 3.5% |
| Magnesium | 13 mg | 3% |
| Manganese | 0.079 mg | 3.5% |
| Phosphorus | 24 mg | 3% |
| Zinc | 0.20 mg | 2% |

# *Daikon*

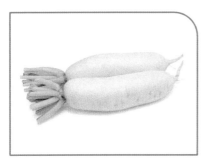

## How to store?

Refrigerate it in a plastic bag for up to 3 days.

## Benefits:

- Detoxifies the Body
- Improves Bone Health
- Inprove digestion
- Anti-inflammatory Agent
- Improves Bone Health

## NUTRITIONAL RATIO

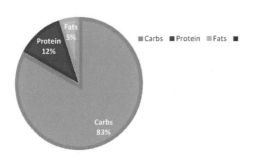

■ Carbs ■ Protein ■ Fats ■

### Nutrition Values for 100g

**Energy:** 16 Kcal

**Carbohydrate:** 3.40 g

**Protein:** 0.68 g

**Total fat:** 0.10 g

**Dietary fiber:** 1.6 g

| Vitamin | Value | RDA % |
|---|---|---|
| Vitamin A | 7 IU | 97% |
| Vitamin C | 14.8 mg | 70.5% |
| Vitamin K | 1.3 µg | 950% |
| Folates | 25 µg | 21% |
| Niancin | 0.254 mg | 4% |
| Pyridoxine | 0.071 mg | 15% |
| Riboflavin | 0.039 mg | 12% |

| Minerals | Value | RDA% |
|---|---|---|
| Calcium | 25 mg | 2.5% |
| Copper | 0.050 mg | 5% |
| Iron | 0.34 mg | 4% |
| Magnesium | 10 mg | 2.5% |
| Manganese | 0.069 mg | 2.5% |
| Zinc | 0.28 mg | 2% |

# *Dandelion Greens*

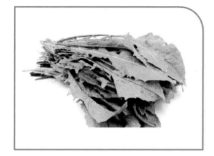

### How to store?

Leaves should be rinsed, dried thoroughly, and stored in an open plastic bag. They'll keep for a few days in the fridge.

### Benefits:

- Detoxify the body
- Inprove digestion
- lower blood pressure
- Prevents Atherosclerosis

## NUTRITIONAL RATIO

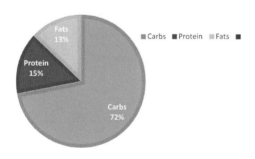

Carbs | Protein | Fats

Fats 13%
Protein 15%
Carbs 72%

### Nutrition Values for 100g

**Energy:** 45 Kcal

**Carbohydrate:** 9.20 g

**Protein:** 2.70 g

**Total fat:** 0.70 g

**Dietary fiber:** 3.50 g

| Vitamin | Value | RDA % |
|---|---|---|
| Vitamin A | 10161 IU | 338% |
| Vitamin C | 35 mg | 58% |
| Vitamin E | 3.44 mg | 23% |
| Vitamin K | 778.4 µg | 649% |
| Folates | 27 µg | 7% |
| Niacin | 0.806 mg | 5% |
| Pantothenic acid | 0.084 mg | 1.5% |
| Pyridoxine | 0.251 mg | 19% |
| Riboflavin | 0.260 mg | 20% |
| Thiamin | 0.190 mg | 17% |

| Minerals | Value | RDA% |
|---|---|---|
| Calcium | 187 mg | 19% |
| Iron | 3.10 mg | 39% |
| Magnesium | 36 mg | 9% |
| Manganese | 0.342 mg | 15% |
| Phosphorus | 66 mg | 9% |
| Selenium | 0.5 mg | 1% |
| Zinc | 0.41 mg | 4% |

# *Edamame, Soybeans*

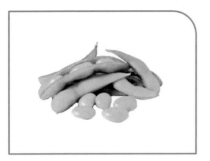

## How to store?

Refrigerate unwashed and covered for up to 3 days.

## Benefits:

- Improve Circulation
- Inprove digestion
- Helps to prevent heart attacks
- Prevent Birth Defects
- Prevents Atherosclerosis

## NUTRITIONAL RATIO

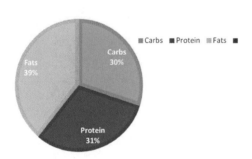

### Nutrition Values for 100g

**Energy:** 109 Kcal

**Carbohydrate:** 7.61 g

**Protein:** 11.22 g

**Total fat:** 4.73 g

**Dietary fiber:** 4.8 g

| Vitamin | Value | RDA % |
|---|---|---|
| Vitamin A | 0 IU | 0% |
| Vitamin C | 9.7 mg | 16% |
| Vitamin E | 0.72 mg | 5% |
| Vitamin K | 31.4 µg | 26% |
| Folates | 303µg | 76% |
| Niancin | 0.925 mg | 6% |
| Pantothenic acid | 0.535 mg | 11% |
| Pyridoxine | 0.135 mg | 10% |
| Riboflavin | 0.265 mg | 20% |
| Thiamin | 0.150 mg | 12.5% |

| Minerals | Value | RDA% |
|---|---|---|
| Calcium | 60 mg | 6% |
| Copper | 0.324 mg | 36% |
| Iron | 2.11 mg | 26% |
| Magnesium | 224 mg | 56% |
| Manganese | 1.672 mg | 73% |
| Phosphorus | 161 mg | 23% |
| Zinc | 1.32 mg | 12% |

## *Eggplant*

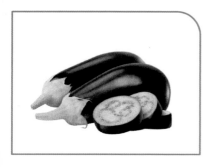

### How to store?

Refrigerate unwashed covered for up to five days.

### Benefits:

- Aid in Digestion
- Improve Bone Health
- Prevent Anemia
- Improve Brain Function
- Reduces risk of anemia

## NUTRITIONAL RATIO

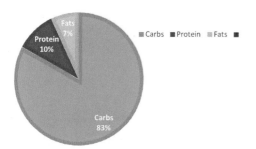

■ Carbs ■ Protein ■ Fats ■

### Nutrition Values for 100g

**Energy:** 24 Kcal

**Carbohydrate:** 5.7 g

**Protein:** 1 g

**Total fat:** 0.19 g

**Dietary fiber:** 3.40 g

| Vitamin | Value | RDA % |
|---|---|---|
| Vitamin A | 27 IU | 1% |
| Vitamin C | 2.2 mg | 3.5% |
| Vitamin E | 0.30 mg | 2% |
| Vitamin K | 3.5 µg | 3% |
| Folates | 22 µg | 5.5% |
| Niancin | 0.649 mg | 4% |
| Pantothenic acid | 0.281 mg | 6% |
| Pyridoxine | 0.084 mg | 6.5% |
| Riboflavin | 0.037 mg | 3% |
| Thiamin | 0..039 mg | 3% |

| Minerals | Value | RDA% |
|---|---|---|
| Calcium | 9 mg | 1% |
| Copper | 0.082 mg | 9% |
| Iron | 0.24 mg | 3% |
| Magnesium | 14 mg | 3.5% |
| Manganese | 0.250 mg | 11% |
| Zinc | 0.16 mg | 1% |

# *Fennel*

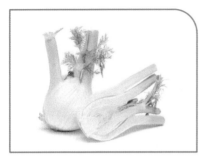

## How to store?

Refrigerate unwashed, covered for 3 to 4 days.

## Benefits:

- Prevents Anemia
- Reduces Heart Diseases
- Treats Constipation
- Regulates Blood Pressure
- Treats Diarrhea & Colic

## NUTRITIONAL RATIO

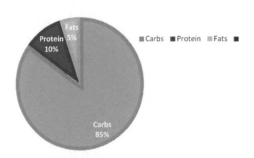

■ Carbs ■ Protein ■ Fats ■

### Nutrition Values for 100g

**Energy:** 31 Kcal

**Carbohydrate:** 7.29 g

**Protein:** 1.24 g

**Total fat:** 0.20 g

**Dietary fiber:** 3.1 g

| Vitamin | Value | RDA % |
|---|---|---|
| Vitamin A | 134 IU | 4.5% |
| Vitamin C | 12 mg | 20% |
| Folates | 27 µg | 7% |
| Niancin | 0.640 mg | 4% |
| Pantothenic acid | 0.232 mg | 5% |
| Pyridoxine | 0.047 mg | 5% |
| Riboflavin | 0.032 mg | 2.5% |
| Thiamin | 0..010 mg | 1% |

| Minerals | Value | RDA% |
|---|---|---|
| Calcium | 49 mg | 5% |
| Copper | 0.066 mg | 7% |
| Iron | 0.73 mg | 9% |
| Magnesium | 17 mg | 4% |
| Manganese | 0.191 mg | 1% |
| Phosphorus | 50 mg | 9% |
| Selenium | 0.7 µg | 1% |
| Zinc | 0.20 mg | 2% |

# *Fiddleheads*

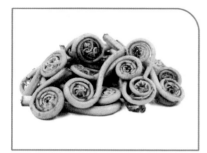

### How to store?

Fresh fiddleheads keep well cooled and tightly wrapped in plastic wrap to prevent drying out for up to 3 days. After blanching and freezing, fiddleheads will keep for several months in the freezer.

### Benefits:

- Fight infections
- Rich in antioxidants
- Maintai blood pressure
- Helps with weight loss

## NUTRITIONAL RATIO

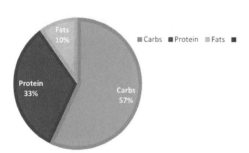

Carbs ■ Protein ■ Fats ■

Fats 10%
Protein 33%
Carbs 57%

## Nutrition Values for 100g

**Energy:** 34 Kcal

**Carbohydrate:** 5.54 g

**Protein:** 4.55 g

**Total fat:** 0.40 g

**Dietary fiber:** 0 g

| Vitamin | Value | RDA % |
|---------|-------|-------|
| Vitamin A | 3617 IU | 120.5% |
| Vitamin C | 26.6 mg | 44% |
| Niancin | 4.980 mg | 31% |
| Riboflavin | 0.210 mg | 16% |
| Thiamin | 0.020 mg | 1.5% |

| Minerals | Value | RDA% |
|----------|-------|------|
| Calcium | 32 mg | 3% |
| Copper | 0.320 mg | 35.5% |
| Iron | 1.31 mg | 16% |
| Magnesium | 34 mg | 8.5% |
| Manganese | 0.510 mg | 22% |
| Selenium | 0.7 µg | 1% |
| Zinc | 0.83 mg | 7.5% |

# *Ginger Root*

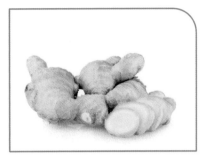

<u>How to store?</u>

Keep it dry in the refrigerator for up to 2 to 3 weeks.

<u>Benefits:</u>

- Aids in Digestion
- Relieves Nausea
- Liver Protection
- Removes Excess Gas
- Reduces Arthritis Pain

## NUTRITIONAL RATIO

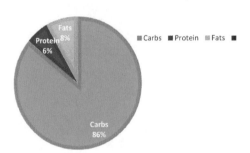

■ Carbs ■ Protein ■ Fats ■

### Nutrition Values for 100g

**Energy:** 80 Kcal

**Carbohydrate:** 17.77 g

**Protein:** 1.82 g

**Total fat:** 0.75 g

**Dietary fiber:** 2.0 g

| Vitamin | Value | RDA % |
|---|---|---|
| Vitamin A | 0 IU | 0% |
| Vitamin C | 5 mg | 8% |
| Vitamin E | 0.26 mg | 1.5% |
| Vitamin K | 0.1 µg | 0% |
| Folates | 11 µg | 3% |
| Niancin | 0.750 mg | 4.5% |
| Pantothenic acid | 0.203 mg | 4% |
| Pyridoxine | 0.160 mg | 12% |

| Minerals | Value | RDA% |
|---|---|---|
| Calcium | 16 mg | 1.6% |
| Copper | 0.226 mg | 25% |
| Iron | 0.60 mg | 7.5% |
| Magnesium | 43 mg | 11% |
| Manganese | 0.229 mg | 10% |
| Phosphorus | 34 mg | 5% |
| Zinc | 0.34 mg | 3% |

# *Horseradish*

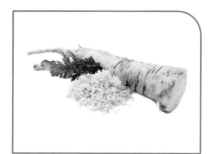

## How to store?

Wrap stems in a damp paper towel and store in the refrigerator for several weeks.

## Benefits:

- Improves Bone Health
- Inprove digestion
- Improves Respiratory Conditions
- Lowers Blood Pressure
- Antibacterial Agent

## NUTRITIONAL RATIO

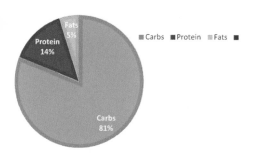

■ Carbs ■ Protein ■ Fats ■

### Nutrition Values for 100g

**Energy:** 48 Kcal

**Carbohydrate:** 11.29 g

**Protein:** 1.18 g

**Total fat:** 0.69 g

**Dietary fiber:** 3.3 g

| Vitamin | Value | RDA % |
|---|---|---|
| Vitamin A | 2 IU | <1% |
| Vitamin C | 24.9 mg | 41% |
| Folates | 57 µg | 14% |
| Niancin | 0.386 mg | 2.5% |
| Pantothenic acid | 0.093 mg | 2% |
| Pyridoxine | 0.073 mg | 6% |
| Riboflavin | 0.024 mg | 2% |
| Thiamin | 0..008 mg | <1% |

| Minerals | Value | RDA% |
|---|---|---|
| Calcium | 56 mg | 6% |
| Copper | 0.058 mg | 6% |
| Iron | 0.42 mg | 5% |
| Magnesium | 27 mg | 7% |
| Manganese | 0.126 mg | 5.5% |
| Phosphorus | 31 mg | 4.5% |
| Zinc | 0.83 mg | 8% |

# *Jicama*

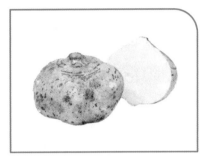

## How to store?

Place in a cool dry place or refrigerate uncovered up to 3 weeks. Once cut, refrigerate covered, up to 1 week.

## Benefits:

- Boosts Immune System
- Strengthens Bones
- Inprove digestion
- Prevents heart diseases
- Improves Blood Circulation

## NUTRITIONAL RATIO

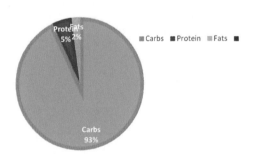

■ Carbs  ■ Protein  ■ Fats  ■

Proteins 5%  Fats 2%

Carbs 93%

### Nutrition Values for 100g

**Energy:** 38 Kcal

**Carbohydrate:** 8.82 g

**Protein:** 0.72 g

**Total fat:** 0.19 g

**Dietary fiber:** 4.9 g

| Vitamin | Value | RDA % |
|---|---|---|
| Vitamin A | 21 IU | 1% |
| Vitamin C | 20.2 mg | 34% |
| Vitamin E | 0.46 mg | 3% |
| Vitamin K | 0.3 µg | <1% |
| Folates | 12 µg | 3% |
| Niancin | 0.200 mg | 1.5% |
| Pantothenic acid | 0.135 mg | 3% |
| Pyridoxine | 0.042 mg | 3% |
| Riboflavin | 0.029 mg | 2% |
| Thiamin | 0..020 mg | 2% |

| Minerals | Value | RDA% |
|---|---|---|
| Calcium | 12 mg | 1% |
| Copper | 0.048 mg | 5% |
| Iron | 0.60 mg | 7% |
| Magnesium | 12 mg | 3% |
| Manganese | 0.60 mg | 3% |
| Zinc | 0.16 mg | 1% |

# *Kale*

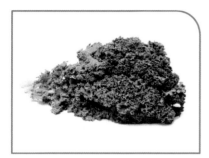

### How to store?

Store kale in a plastic bag in the coldest part of the fridge for 3-5 days.

### Benefits:

- Hair & Skin Care
- Reduces Inflammation
- Lowers Blood Pressure
- Improves Digestion
- Improve vision

## NUTRITIONAL RATIO

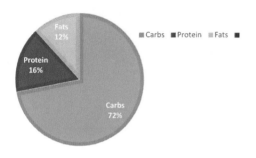

Carbs · Protein · Fats ·

Fats 12%
Protein 16%
Carbs 72%

### Nutrition Values for 100g

**Energy:** 35 Kcal

**Carbohydrate:** 4.42 g

**Protein:** 2.92 g

**Total fat:** 1.49 g

**Dietary fiber:** 4.1 g

| Vitamin | Value | RDA % |
|---|---|---|
| Vitamin A | 4812 IU | 160% |
| Vitamin C | 93.4 mg | 156% |
| Vitamin K | 389.6 µg | 325% |
| Folates | 62 µg | 15.5% |
| Niancin | 1.180 mg | 7% |
| Pantothenic acid | 0.370 mg | 7% |
| Pyridoxine | 0.147 mg | 11% |
| Riboflavin | 0.347 mg | 27% |
| Thiamin | 0.113 mg | 9% |

| Minerals | Value | RDA% |
|---|---|---|
| Calcium | 245 mg | 25% |
| Copper | 0.053 mg | 6% |
| Iron | 1.60 mg | 20% |
| Magnesium | 33 mg | 8% |
| Manganese | 0.920 mg | 40% |
| Phosphorus | 55 mg | 8% |
| Selenium | 0.9 µg | 1.6% |
| Zinc | 0.39 mg | 3.5% |

# *Kohlrabi*

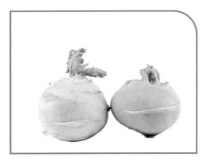

## How to store?

Cut off leaves and refrigerate bulbs unwashed, covered for up to 1 week. Store leaves covered and refrigerated a few days.

## Benefits:

- Boosts Energy Level
- Inprove digestion
- Regulates Blood Pressure
- Eye Care

## NUTRITIONAL RATIO

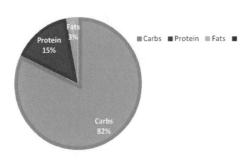

■ Carbs ■ Protein ■ Fats ■

### Nutrition Values for 100g

**Energy:** 27 Kcal

**Carbohydrate:** 6.20 g

**Protein:** 1.70 g

**Total fat:** 0.10 g

**Dietary fiber:** 3.6 g

| Vitamin | Value | RDA % |
|---|---|---|
| Vitamin A | 36 IU | 1% |
| Vitamin C | 62 mg | 102% |
| Vitamin K | 0.1 µg | <1% |
| Folates | 16 µg | 4% |
| Niancin | 0.400 mg | 2.5% |
| Pantothenic acid | 0.165 mg | 3% |
| Pyridoxine | 0.150 mg | 11.5% |
| Riboflavin | 0.020 mg | 1.5% |
| Thiamin | 0..050 mg | 4% |

| Minerals | Value | RDA% |
|---|---|---|
| Calcium | 24 mg | 2.5% |
| Copper | 0.129 mg | 14% |
| Iron | 0.40 mg | 5% |
| Magnesium | 19 mg | 5% |
| Manganese | 0.139 mg | 6% |
| Phosphorus | 46 mg | 6.5% |
| Selenium | 0.7 µg | 1% |
| Zinc | 0.03 mg | <1% |

# *Leeks*

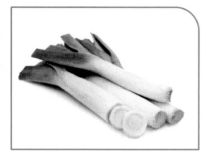

### How to store?

Refrigerate unwashed leeks in plastic bag for up to 2 weeks. Rinse before using.

### Benefits:

- Detoxifies the skin
- Aids Digestion
- Promotes Hair Growth
- Improves Vision
- Protects Blood Vessels

## NUTRITIONAL RATIO

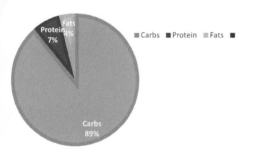

Carbs ■ Protein ■ Fats ■

Protein 7%
Fats 4%
Carbs 89%

### Nutrition Values for 100g

**Energy:** 61 Kcal

**Carbohydrate:** 14.15 g

**Protein:** 1.5 g

**Total fat:** 0.30 g

**Dietary fiber:** 1.8 g

| Vitamin | Value | RDA % |
|---|---|---|
| Vitamin A | 1667 IU | 55% |
| Vitamin C | 12 mg | 20% |
| Vitamin E | 0.92 mg | 6% |
| Vitamin K | 47 µg | 39% |
| Folates | 64 µg | 16% |
| Niacin | 0.400 mg | 2.5% |
| Pantothenic acid | 0.140 mg | 3% |
| Pyridoxine | 0.233 mg | 18% |
| Riboflavin | 0.030 mg | 2% |
| Thiamin | 0.060 mg | 5% |

| Minerals | Value | RDA% |
|---|---|---|
| Calcium | 59 mg | 6% |
| Copper | 0.120 mg | 13% |
| Iron | 2.10 mg | 26% |
| Magnesium | 28 mg | 7% |
| Manganese | 0.481 mg | 2% |
| Phosphorus | 35 mg | 5% |
| Selenium | 1 µg | 2% |
| Zinc | 1.2 mg | 11% |

# *Lettuce (Iceberg)*

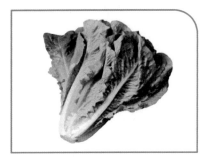

### How to store?

Remove core, rinse, dry well. Wrap in towel, store in airtight container, refrigerate for up to five days.

### Benefits:

• Helps in digestion

• Prevents birth defects

• Lowers Cholesterol Levels

• Prevents anemia

• Protects the heart

## NUTRITIONAL RATIO

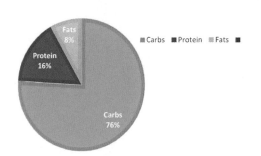

■ Carbs  ■ Protein  ■ Fats  ■

Fats 8%
Protein 16%
Carbs 76%

### Nutrition Values for 100g

**Energy:** 14 Kcal

**Carbohydrate:** 3.2 g

**Protein:** 0.9 g

**Total fat:** 0.1 g

**Dietary fiber:** 1.2 g

| Vitamin | Value | RDA % |
|---|---|---|
| Vitamin A | 3790 IU | 76% |
| Vitamin C | 21.1 mg | 35% |
| Vitamin E | 1.4 mg | 7% |
| Vitamin K | 182 µg | 227% |
| Folates | 219 µg | 55% |
| Niancin | 0.9 mg | 5% |
| Pantothenic acid | 0.7 mg | 7% |
| Riboflavin | 0.2 mg | 11% |
| Thiamin | 0.3 mg | 21% |

| Minerals | Value | RDA% |
|---|---|---|
| Calcium | 136 mg | 14% |
| Copper | 0.2 mg | 9% |
| Iron | 3.1 mg | 17% |
| Magnesium | 52.9 mg | 13% |
| Manganese | 0.9 mg | 47% |
| Phosphorus | 151 mg | 15% |
| Selenium | 0.8 µg | 1% |
| Zinc | 1.1 mg | 8% |

# *Lettuce (Leaf)*

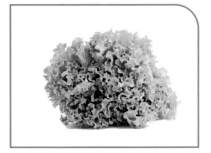

### How to store?

Rinse, dry well. Wrap in towel, store in airtight container, refrigerate for up to five days.

### Benefits:

- Anti-inflammatory Agent
- Antioxidant Agent
- Induces Sleep
- Controls Anxiety
- Lowers Cholesterol Levels

## NUTRITIONAL RATIO

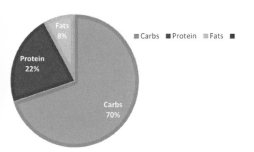

■ Carbs   ■ Protein   ■ Fats   ■

### Nutrition Values for 100g

**Energy:** 15 Kcal

**Carbohydrate:** 2.87 g

**Protein:** 1.36 g

**Total fat:** 0.15 g

**Dietary fiber:** 1.3 g

| Vitamin | Value | RDA % |
|---|---|---|
| Vitamin A | 7405 IU | 247% |
| Vitamin C | 9.2 mg | 15% |
| Vitamin E | 0.29 mg | 2% |
| Vitamin K | 126.3 µg | 105% |
| Folates | 38 µg | 9.5% |
| Niacin | 0.375 mg | 2% |
| Pantothenic acid | 0.134 mg | 2.5% |
| Pyridoxine | 0.090 mg | 7% |
| Riboflavin | 0.080 mg | 6% |
| Thiamin | 0..070 mg | 6% |

| Minerals | Value | RDA% |
|---|---|---|
| Calcium | 36 mg | 3.5% |
| Copper | 0.029 mg | 3% |
| Iron | 0.86 mg | 10% |
| Magnesium | 13 mg | 3% |
| Manganese | 0250 mg | 11% |
| Phosphorus | 29 mg | 4% |
| Zinc | 0.18 mg | 1.5% |

# Lettuce (Romaine)

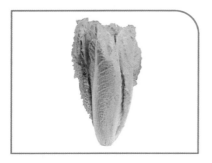

### How to store?

Rinse, dry well. Wrap in towel, store in airtight container, refrigerate for up to five days.

### Benefits:

- Prevents Bone Loss
- Prevents Signs of Aging
- Improve vision
- Improves Digestion
- Treats Insomnia

## NUTRITIONAL RATIO

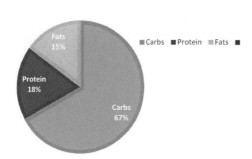

■ Carbs ■ Protein ■ Fats ■

### Nutrition Values for 100g

**Energy:** 17 Kcal

**Carbohydrate:** 3.3 g

**Protein:** 1.2 g

**Total fat:** 0.3 g

**Dietary fiber:** 2.1 g

| Vitamin | Value | RDA % |
|---|---|---|
| Vitamin A | 8711 IU | 174% |
| Vitamin C | 24 mg | 40% |
| Vitamin E | 0.1 mg | 1% |
| Vitamin K | 103 µg | 128% |
| Folates | 136 µg | 34% |
| Niacin | 0.3 mg | 2% |
| Pantothenic acid | 0.1 mg | 1% |
| Riboflavin | 0.1 mg | 4% |
| Thiamin | 0.1 mg | 5% |

| Minerals | Value | RDA% |
|---|---|---|
| Calcium | 33 mg | 3% |
| Iron | 1.0 mg | 5% |
| Magnesium | 14 mg | 3% |
| Manganese | 0.2 mg | 8% |
| Phosphorus | 30 mg | 3% |
| Selenium | 0.4 µg | 1% |
| Zinc | 0.2 mg | 2% |

# *Mushrooms*

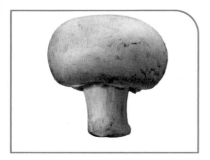

### How to store?

Store mushrooms in your refrigerator crisper where they can benefit from cool air circulation. Keep partially covered to prevent them from drying out, but never store packaged fresh mushrooms without venting. Paper bags are a good storage option. Use fresh mushrooms within 3 days.

### Benefits:

- Lower Cholesterol
- Prevent Diabetes
- Lower Blood Pressure
- Increase Iron Absorption

## NUTRITIONAL RATIO

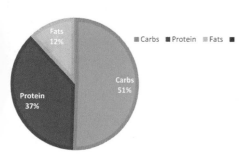

■ Carbs ■ Protein ■ Fats ■

Fats 12%
Carbs 51%
Protein 37%

### Nutrition Values for 100g

**Energy:** 22 Kcal

**Carbohydrate:** 3.26 g

**Protein:** 2.18 g

**Total fat:** 0.34 g

**Dietary fiber:** 1 g

| Vitamin | Value | RDA % |
|---|---|---|
| Vitamin C | 2.1 mg | 3.5% |
| Vitamin D | 7 IU | 1% |
| Folates | 17 µg | 4% |
| Niacin | 3.607 mg | 23% |
| Pantothenic acid | 1.497 mg | 27% |
| Pyridoxine | 0.104 mg | 8% |
| Riboflavin | 0.402 mg | 31% |
| Thiamin | 0.81 mg | 7% |

| Minerals | Value | RDA% |
|---|---|---|
| Calcium | 3 mg | <1% |
| Copper | 0.318 mg | 35% |
| Iron | 0.50 mg | 6% |
| Magnesium | 9 mg | 2% |
| Manganese | 0.047 mg | <1% |
| Phosphorus | 86 mg | 12% |
| Selenium | 9.3 µg | 17% |
| Zinc | 0.52 mg | 15% |

# *Mustard Greens*

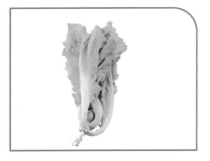

### How to store?

Discard any bruised or yellow leaves and remove any bands or ties that hold bunches together. Gently wrap unwashed mustard greens in paper towels and store loosely in plastic bags. Store for up to 5 days.

### Benefits:

• anti-inflammatory benefits    • improve brain health

• Inprove eye health    • improve digestion

## NUTRITIONAL RATIO

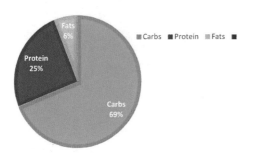

■ Carbs  ■ Protein  ■ Fats  ■

### Nutrition Values for 100g

**Energy:** 27 Kcal

**Carbohydrate:** 4.67 g

**Protein:** 2.86 g

**Total fat:** 0.42 g

**Dietary fiber:** 3.20 g

| Vitamin | Value | RDA % |
|---|---|---|
| Vitamin A | 3024 IU | 101% |
| Vitamin C | 70 mg | 117% |
| Vitamin E | 0 | 0% |
| Vitamin K | 257.5 µg | 215% |
| Folates | 12 µg | 3% |
| Niancin | 0.800 mg | 5% |
| Pantothenic acid | 0.210 mg | 5% |
| Pyridoxine | 0.180 mg | 14% |
| Riboflavin | 0.110 mg | 8% |
| Thiamin | 0..080 mg | 7% |

| Minerals | Value | RDA% |
|---|---|---|
| Calcium | 115 mg | 11.5% |
| Copper | 0.165 mg | 18% |
| Iron | 1.64 mg | 20% |
| Magnesium | 32 mg | 8% |
| Manganese | 0.480 mg | 21% |
| Selenium | 0.9 µg | 1.5% |
| Zinc | 0.25 mg | 2% |

*Okra*

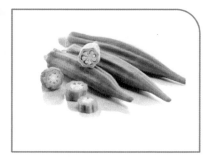

### How to store?

Refrigerate unwashed covered for up to 3 days.

### Benefits:

- Reduces Fatigue
- Inprove digestion
- Anti-stress Effect
- Diabetes Management
- Lowers Cholesterol Levels

## NUTRITIONAL RATIO

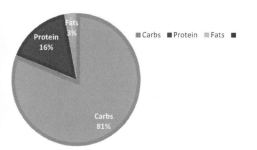

■ Carbs ■ Protein ■ Fats ■

## Nutrition Values for 100g

**Energy:** 33 Kcal

**Carbohydrate:** 7.03 g

**Protein:** 2.0 g

**Total fat:** 0.1 g

**Dietary fiber:** 9 g

| Vitamin | Value | RDA % |
|---|---|---|
| Vitamin A | 375 IU | 12.5% |
| Vitamin C | 21.1 mg | 2.5% |
| Vitamin E | 0.36 mg | 36% |
| Vitamin K | 53 µg | 44% |
| Folates | 88 µg | 22% |
| Niacin | 1.000 mg | 6% |
| Pantothenic acid | 0.245 mg | 5% |
| Pyridoxine | 0.215 mg | 16.5% |
| Riboflavin | 0.060 mg | 4.5% |
| Thiamin | 0..200 mg | 17% |

| Minerals | Value | RDA% |
|---|---|---|
| Calcium | 81 mg | 8% |
| Copper | 0.094 mg | 10% |
| Iron | 0.80 mg | 10% |
| Magnesium | 57 mg | 14% |
| Manganese | 0.990 mg | 43% |
| Phosphorus | 63 mg | 9% |
| Selenium | 0.7 µg | 1% |
| Zinc | 0.60 mg | 5.5% |

# *Onion (Red)*

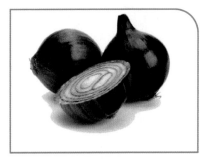

## How to store?

Keep onions in a dark, cool location. o not store next to potatoes since both vegetables give off a gas that will cause the other vegetable to rot. Once cut, wrap the onion in plastic, store in the refrigerator and use within a couple of days.

## Benefits:

• Detoxify the body     • Reduce blood pressre

## NUTRITIONAL RATIO

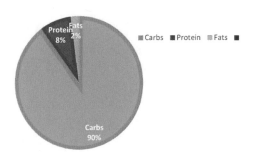

■ Carbs ■ Protein ■ Fats ■

Protein 8%   Fats 2%   Carbs 90%

### Nutrition Values for 100g

**Energy: 40 Kcal**

**Carbohydrate: 9.34 g**

**Protein: 1.10 g**

**Total fat: 0.10 g**

**Dietary fiber: 1.7 g**

| Vitamin | Value | RDA % |
|---|---|---|
| Vitamin A | 2 IU | 0% |
| Vitamin C | 7.4 mg | 12% |
| Vitamin K | 0.02 µg | 0% |
| Folates | 19 µg | 5% |
| Niancin | 0.116 mg | 1% |
| Pantothenic acid | 0.123 mg | 2.5% |
| Pyridoxine | 0.120 mg | 9% |
| Riboflavin | 0.027 mg | 2% |
| Thiamin | 0..046 mg | 4% |

| Minerals | Value | RDA% |
|---|---|---|
| Calcium | 23 mg | 2% |
| Copper | 0.039 mg | 4% |
| Iron | 0.21 mg | 3% |
| Magnesium | 10 mg | 2.5% |
| Manganese | 0.129 mg | 5.5% |
| Phosphorus | 29 mg | 4% |
| Zinc | 0.17 mg | 1.5% |

# *Onion*

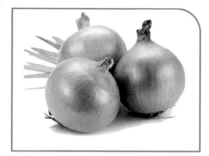

### How to store?

Keep uncovered in a dry dark place for up to two months or at room temperature for up to three weeks. Cover cut portions and refrigerate for up to four days.

### Benefits:

- Oral Care
- Treat Cough
- Manage Diabetes
- Treat Anemia

## NUTRITIONAL RATIO

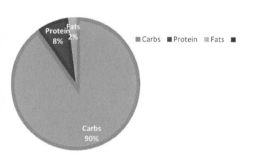

Carbs ■ Protein ■ Fats ■

Protein 8%
Fats 2%
Carbs 90%

### Nutrition Values for 100g

**Energy:** 40 Kcal

**Carbohydrate:** 9.34 g

**Protein:** 1.10 g

**Total fat:** 0.10 g

**Dietary fiber:** 1.7 g

| Vitamin | Value | RDA % |
|---|---|---|
| Vitamin A | 2 IU | 0% |
| Vitamin C | 7.4 mg | 12% |
| Vitamin K | 0.02 µg | 0% |
| Folates | 19 µg | 5% |
| Niancin | 0.116 mg | 1% |
| Pantothenic acid | 0.123 mg | 2.5% |
| Pyridoxine | 0.120 mg | 9% |
| Riboflavin | 0.027 mg | 2% |
| Thiamin | 0..046 mg | 4% |

| Minerals | Value | RDA% |
|---|---|---|
| Calcium | 23 mg | 2% |
| Copper | 0.039 mg | 4% |
| Iron | 0.21 mg | 3% |
| Magnesium | 10 mg | 2.5% |
| Manganese | 0.129 mg | 5.5% |
| Phosphorus | 29 mg | 4% |
| Zinc | 0.17 mg | 1.5% |

# *Parsnip*

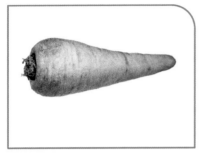

## How to store?

Refrigerate unwashed, covered for up to 10 days.

## Benefits:

- Improve Heart Health
- Oral Health
- Aid Digestion
- Reduce Birth Defects
- Enhance Vision

## NUTRITIONAL RATIO

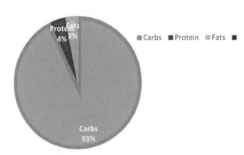

■ Carbs  ■ Protein  ■ Fats  ■

### Nutrition Values for 100g

**Energy:** 75 Kcal

**Carbohydrate:** 17.99 g

**Protein:** 1.20 g

**Total fat:** 0.30 g

**Dietary fiber:** 4.9 g

| Vitamin | Value | RDA % |
|---|---|---|
| Vitamin A | 0 IU | 97% |
| Vitamin C | 17 mg | 70.5% |
| Vitamin K | 22.5 µg | 950% |
| Folates | 67 µg | 21% |
| Niacin | 0.700 mg | 4% |
| Pantothenic acid | 0.600 mg | 1% |
| Pyridoxine | 0.90 mg | 15% |
| Riboflavin | 0.050 mg | 12% |
| Thiamin | 0..090 mg | 2% |

| Minerals | Value | RDA% |
|---|---|---|
| Calcium | 36 mg | 3.5% |
| Copper | 0.120 mg | 13% |
| Iron | 0.59 mg | 7.5% |
| Magnesium | 29 mg | 7% |
| Manganese | 0.560 mg | 24% |
| Phosphorus | 71 mg | 10% |
| Selenium | 1.8 µg | 3% |
| Zinc | 0.59 mg | 5% |

# *Peas (Green)*

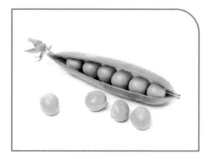

## How to store?

Refrigerate peas in a perforated plastic bag for 3-5 days.

## Benefits:

- Anti-Aging
- Aids liver function
- Regulates blood sugar
- Immune booster
- Prevents stomach cancer

## NUTRITIONAL RATIO

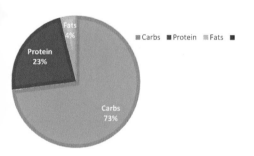

■ Carbs ■ Protein ■ Fats ■

### Nutrition Values for 100g

**Energy:** 81 Kcal

**Carbohydrate:** 14.45 g

**Protein:** 5.42 g

**Total fat:** 0.40 g

**Dietary fiber:** 5.1 g

| Vitamin | Value | RDA % |
|---|---|---|
| Vitamin A | 765 IU | 25.5% |
| Vitamin C | 40 mg | 67% |
| Vitamin E | 0.13 mg | 1 |
| Vitamin K | 24.8 µg | 21% |
| Folates | 65 µg | 16% |
| Niacin | 2.090 mg | 13% |
| Pantothenic acid | 0.104 mg | 2% |
| Pyridoxine | 0.169 mg | 13% |
| Riboflavin | 0.132 mg | 10% |
| Thiamin | 0..266 mg | 22% |

| Minerals | Value | RDA% |
|---|---|---|
| Calcium | 25 mg | 2.5% |
| Copper | 0.176 mg | 20% |
| Iron | 1.47 mg | 18% |
| Magnesium | 33 mg | 8% |
| Manganese | 0.410 mg | 18% |
| Selenium | 1.8 µg | 3% |
| Zinc | 1.24 mg | 11% |

# *Pepper (Green)*

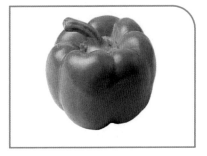

### How to store?

Cover, refrigerate unwashed for up to one week.

### Benefits:

- Boost immune system
- Strengthens the bone
- Delay aging process
- Antioxydant agent
- Fight colon cance

## NUTRITIONAL RATIO

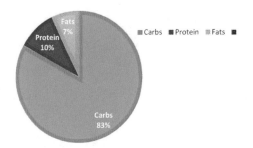

Carbs ■ Protein ■ Fats ■

### Nutrition Values for 100g

**Energy:** 31 Kcal

**Carbohydrate:** 6.03 g

**Protein:** 0.99 g

**Total fat:** 0.30 g

**Dietary fiber:** 2.1 g

| Vitamin | Value | RDA % |
|---------|-------|-------|
| Vitamin A | 3131 IU | 101% |
| Vitamin C | 127.7 mg | 213% |
| Vitamin E | 1.58 mg | 11% |
| Vitamin K | 4.9 àµg | 4% |
| Folates | 46 µg | 12% |
| Niancin | 0.979 mg | 6% |
| Pyridoxine | 0.291 mg | 22% |
| Riboflavin | 0.058 mg | 6.5% |
| Thiamin | 0..054 mg | 4.5% |

| Minerals | Value | RDA% |
|----------|-------|------|
| Calcium | 7 mg | 1% |
| Copper | 0.017 mg | 2% |
| Iron | 0.43 mg | 5% |
| Magnesium | 12 mg | 3% |
| Manganese | 0.112 mg | 5% |
| Phosphorus | 26 mg | 4% |
| Selenium | 0.1 µg | <1% |

# *Pepper (Red, Sweet)*

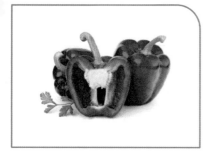

### How to store?

Cover, refrigerate unwashed for up to one week.

### Benefits:

- Boost immune system
- Strengthens the bone
- Delay aging process
- Antioxydant agent
- Fight colon cance

## NUTRITIONAL RATIO

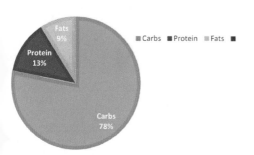

### Nutrition Values for 100g

**Energy:** 31 Kcal

**Carbohydrate:** 6.03 g

**Protein:** 0.99 g

**Total fat:** 0.30 g

**Dietary fiber:** 2.1 g

| Vitamin | Value | RDA % |
|---|---|---|
| Vitamin A | 3131 IU | 101% |
| Vitamin C | 127.7 mg | 213% |
| Vitamin E | 1.58 mg | 11% |
| Vitamin K | 4.9 àµg | 4% |
| Folates | 46 µg | 12% |
| Niancin | 0.979 mg | 6% |
| Pyridoxine | 0.291 mg | 22% |
| Riboflavin | 0.058 mg | 6.5% |
| Thiamin | 0..054 mg | 4.5% |

| Minerals | Value | RDA% |
|---|---|---|
| Calcium | 7 mg | 1% |
| Copper | 0.017 mg | 2% |
| Iron | 0.43 mg | 5% |
| Magnesium | 12 mg | 3% |
| Manganese | 0.112 mg | 5% |
| Phosphorus | 26 mg | 4% |
| Selenium | 0.1 µg | <1% |
| Zinc | 0.25 mg | 2% |

# Potatoes (Red)

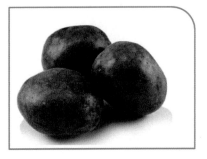

### How to store?

Keep in a cool, dry, dark, ventilated place for up to two months or keep at room temperature for up to one week. Do not refrigerate except new potatoes for up to one week.

### Benefits:

- Promote Weight Gain
- Skin Care
- Treat Kidney Stones
- Treat Diarrhea

## NUTRITIONAL RATIO

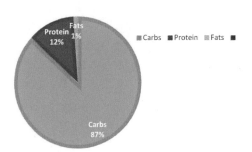

| | | |
|---|---|---|
| ■ Carbs | ■ Protein | ■ Fats ■ |

### Nutrition Values for 100g

**Energy:** 77 Kcal

**Carbohydrate:** 17.49 g

**Protein:** 2.05 g

**Total fat:** 0.10 g

**Dietary fiber:** 2.1 g

| Vitamin | Value | RDA % |
|---|---|---|
| Vitamin A | 2 IU | <1% |
| Vitamin C | 19.7 mg | 33% |
| Vitamin K | 2 mcg | 2% |
| Folates | 15 µg | 4% |
| Niancin | 1.061 mg | 6% |
| Pantothenic acid | 0.279 mg | 6% |
| Pyridoxine | 0.298 mg | 23% |
| Riboflavin | 0.032 mg | 2.5% |
| Thiamin | 0..081 mg | 7% |

| Minerals | Value | RDA% |
|---|---|---|
| Calcium | 12 mg | 1% |
| Iron | 0.81 mg | 10% |
| Magnesium | 23 mg | 6% |
| Manganese | 0.141 mg | 6% |
| Phosphorus | 57 mg | 8% |
| Zinc | 0.30 mg | 3% |

# *Potatoes (White)*

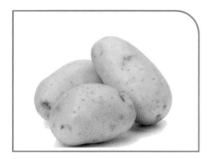

## How to store?

Keep in a cool, dry, dark, ventilated place for up to two months or keep at room temperature for up to one week. Do not refrigerate except new potatoes for up to one week.

## Benefits:

- Promote Weight Gain
- Skin Care
- Treat Kidney Stones
- Treat Diarrhea

### NUTRITIONAL RATIO

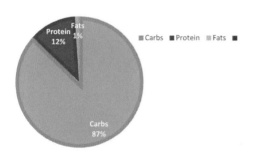

Protein 12%
Fats 1%
Carbs 87%

■ Carbs  ■ Protein  ■ Fats  ■

### Nutrition Values for 100g

**Energy:** 77 Kcal

**Carbohydrate:** 17.49 g

**Protein:** 2.05 g

**Total fat:** 0.10 g

**Dietary fiber:** 2.1 g

| Vitamin | Value | RDA % |
|---|---|---|
| Vitamin A | 2 IU | <1% |
| Vitamin C | 19.7 mg | 33% |
| Vitamin K | 2 mcg | 2% |
| Folates | 15 µg | 4% |
| Niancin | 1.061 mg | 6% |
| Pantothenic acid | 0.279 mg | 6% |
| Pyridoxine | 0.298 mg | 23% |
| Riboflavin | 0.032 mg | 2.5% |
| Thiamin | 0..081 mg | 7% |

| Minerals | Value | RDA% |
|---|---|---|
| Calcium | 12 mg | 1% |
| Iron | 0.81 mg | 10% |
| Magnesium | 23 mg | 6% |
| Manganese | 0.141 mg | 6% |
| Phosphorus | 57 mg | 8% |
| Zinc | 0.30 mg | 3% |

# *Potatoes (Yellow)*

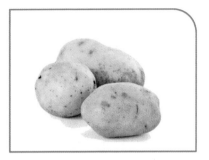

### How to store?

Keep in a cool, dry, dark, ventilated place for up to two months or keep at room temperature for up to one week. Do not refrigerate except new potatoes for up to one week.

### Benefits:

- Promote Weight Gain
- Skin Care
- Treat Kidney Stones
- Treat Diarrhea

## NUTRITIONAL RATIO

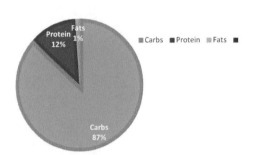

### Nutrition Values for 100g

**Energy:** 77 Kcal

**Carbohydrate:** 17.49 g

**Protein:** 2.05 g

**Total fat:** 0.10 g

**Dietary fiber:** 2.1 g

| Vitamin | Value | RDA % |
|---|---|---|
| Vitamin A | 2 IU | <1% |
| Vitamin C | 19.7 mg | 33% |
| Vitamin K | 2 mcg | 2% |
| Folates | 15 µg | 4% |
| Niancin | 1.061 mg | 6% |
| Pantothenic acid | 0.279 mg | 6% |
| Pyridoxine | 0.298 mg | 23% |
| Riboflavin | 0.032 mg | 2.5% |
| Thiamin | 0..081 mg | 7% |

| Minerals | Value | RDA% |
|---|---|---|
| Calcium | 12 mg | 1% |
| Iron | 0.81 mg | 10% |
| Magnesium | 23 mg | 6% |
| Manganese | 0.141 mg | 6% |
| Phosphorus | 57 mg | 8% |
| Zinc | 0.30 mg | 3% |

# *Pumpkin*

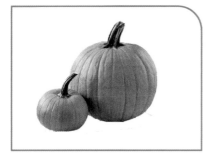

## How to store?

Keep at room temperature for up to one week; do not refrigerate. Refrigerate cut portions up to 5 days.

## Benefits:

- Boosts Immunity
- Increases Fertility
- Protects Vision
- Strengthens Bones
- high levels of antioxidants

## NUTRITIONAL RATIO

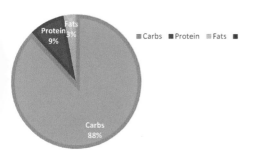

- Carbs ■ Protein ■ Fats ■

Fats 5%
Protein 9%
Carbs 88%

### Nutrition Values for 100g

**Energy:** 26 Kcal

**Carbohydrate:** 6.50 g

**Protein:** 1.0 g

**Total fat:** 0.1 g

**Dietary fiber:** 0.5 g

| Vitamin | Value | RDA % |
|---|---|---|
| Vitamin A | 7384 IU | 246% |
| Vitamin C | 9.0 mg | 15% |
| Vitamin E | 1.06 mg | 7% |
| Vitamin K | 1.1 mcg | 1% |
| Folates | 16 µg | 4% |
| Niacin | 0.600 mg | 4% |
| Pantothenic acid | 0.298 mg | 6% |
| Pyridoxine | 0.061 mg | 5% |
| Riboflavin | 0.110 mg | 8.5% |
| Thiamin | 0..050 mg | 4% |

| Minerals | Value | RDA% |
|---|---|---|
| Calcium | 21 mg | 2% |
| Copper | 0.127 mg | 14% |
| Iron | 0.80 mg | 10% |
| Magnesium | 12 mg | 3% |
| Manganese | 0.125 mg | 0.5% |
| Phosphorus | 44 mg | 5% |
| Selenium | 0.3 mcg | <0.5% |
| Zinc | 0.32 mg | 3% |

# *Radicchio*

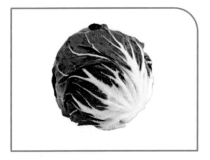

## How to store?

Refrigerate unwashed for no more than 3 days.

## Benefits:

• Detoxify the Body

• lower blood pressure

• High in antioxidants

• Aids eyes health

• Lower bad cholesterol level

## NUTRITIONAL RATIO

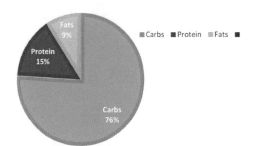

■ Carbs  ■ Protein  ■ Fats  ■

Fats 9%

Protein 15%

Carbs 76%

## Nutrition Values for 100g

**Energy:** 23 Kcal

**Carbohydrate:** 4.48 g

**Protein:** 1.43 g

**Total fat:** 0.25 g

**Dietary fiber:** 0.9 g

| Vitamin | Value | RDA % |
|---|---|---|
| Vitamin A | 27 IU | 1% |
| Vitamin C | 8 mg | 13% |
| Vitamin E | 2.26 mg | 15% |
| Vitamin K | 255.2 µg | 212% |
| Folates | 60 µg | 15% |
| Niancin | 0.255 mg | 1.5% |
| Pantothenic acid | 0.269 mg | 5% |
| Pyridoxine | 0.057 mg | 4% |
| Riboflavin | 0.028 mg | 2% |
| Thiamin | 0..016 mg | 1% |

| Minerals | Value | RDA% |
|---|---|---|
| Calcium | 19 mg | 2% |
| Copper | 0.341 mg | 38% |
| Iron | 0.57 mg | 7% |
| Magnesium | 13 mg | 3% |
| Manganese | 0.138 mg | 6% |
| Phosphorus | 40 mg | 5.5% |
| Selenium | 0.9 µg | 1% |
| Zinc | 0.62 mg | 6% |

# *Radishes*

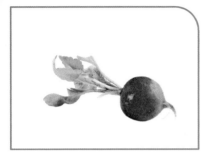

## How to store?

Remove tops. Cover, refrigerate unwashed, for up to one week.

## Benefits:

• Aids in Digestion      • Treats Respiratory Disorders

• Treats Jaundice      • Skin Care

• Treats Urinary Disorders

## NUTRITIONAL RATIO

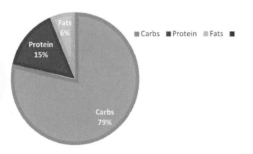

■ Carbs   ■ Protein   ■ Fats ■

### Nutrition Values for 100g

**Energy:** 16 Kcal

**Carbohydrate:** 3.40 g

**Protein:** 0.68 g

**Total fat:** 0.10 g

**Dietary fiber:** 1.6 g

| Vitamin | Value | RDA % |
|---|---|---|
| Vitamin A | 7 IU | <1% |
| Vitamin C | 14.8 mg | 25% |
| Vitamin E | 0 mg | 9% |
| Vitamin K | 1.3 µg | 1% |
| Folates | 25 µg | 6% |
| Niacin | 0.254 mg | 1.5% |
| Pyridoxine | 0.071 mg | 5.5% |
| Riboflavin | 0.039 mg | 3% |

| Minerals | Value | RDA% |
|---|---|---|
| Calcium | 25 mg | 2.5% |
| Copper | 0.050mg | 5% |
| Iron | 0.34 mg | 4% |
| Magnesium | 10 mg | 2.5% |
| Manganese | 0.069 mg | 2.5% |
| Zinc | 0.28 mg | 2% |

# *Rutabaga*

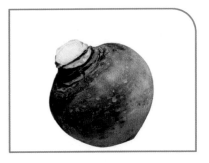

## How to store?

Refrigerate unwashed for up to three weeks or keep at room temperature for up to one week.

## Benefits:

- Boost Immune System
- Boost Metabolism
- Inprove digestion
- Prevent Diabetes
- Prevent Premature Aging

## NUTRITIONAL RATIO

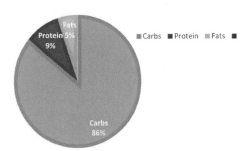

■ Carbs  ■ Protein  ■ Fats  ■

### Nutrition Values for 100g

**Energy:** 37 Kcal

**Carbohydrate:** 8.62 g

**Protein:** 1.06 g

**Total fat:** 0.16 g

**Dietary fiber:** 2.3 g

| Vitamin | Value | RDA % |
|---|---|---|
| Vitamin A | 2 IU | <1% |
| Vitamin C | 25 mg | 42% |
| Folates | 21 µg | 5% |
| Niancin | 0.700 mg | 4% |
| Pantothenic acid | 0.160 mg | 3% |
| Pyridoxine | 0.100 mg | 7.5% |
| Riboflavin | 0.040 mg | 3% |
| Thiamin | 0..090 mg | 7.5% |

| Minerals | Value | RDA% |
|---|---|---|
| Calcium | 43 mg | 4% |
| Copper | 0.032 mg | 3% |
| Iron | 0.44 mg | 5.5% |
| Magnesium | 20 mg | 5% |
| Manganese | 0.131 mg | 6% |
| Zinc | 0.24 mg | 2% |

# *Salsify (Oysterplant)*

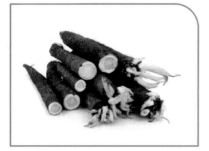

### How to store?

Wrap salsify in a plastic bag and store in the refrigerator for up to two weeks.

### Benefits:

- Improves Circulation
- Improves Hair Health
- Inprove digestion
- Boosts Immune System
- Regulates Blood Pressure

## NUTRITIONAL RATIO

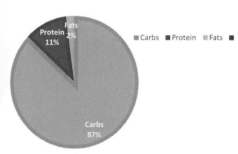

Protein 11%
Fats 2%
Carbs 87%

■ Carbs ■ Protein ■ Fats ■

### Nutrition Values for 100g

**Energy:** 82 Kcal

**Carbohydrate:** 18.60 g

**Protein:** 3.30 g

**Total fat:** 0.20 g

**Dietary fiber:** 3.3 g

| Vitamin | Value | RDA % |
|---|---|---|
| Vitamin A | 0 IU | 0% |
| Vitamin C | 8 mg | 13% |
| Folates | 26 µg | 6.5% |
| Niancin | 0.500 mg | 3% |
| Pantothenic acid | 0.371 mg | 7% |
| Pyridoxine | 0.277 mg | 2% |
| Riboflavin | 0.220 mg | 18% |
| Thiamin | 0.080 mg | 7% |

| Minerals | Value | RDA% |
|---|---|---|
| Calcium | 60 mg | 6% |
| Copper | 0.089 mg | 9% |
| Iron | 0.70 mg | 9% |
| Magnesium | 23 mg | 6% |
| Manganese | 0.268 mg | 12% |
| Phosphorus | 75 mg | 11% |
| Selenium | 0.8 µg | 1% |
| Zinc | 0.38 mg | 3% |

# *Shallots*

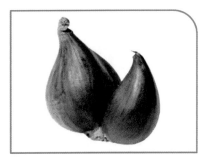

## How to store?

Store whole shallots in a cool, dark, well-ventilated place for use within 4 weeks. Refrigerate cut shallots in an air-tight container for use within 2-3 days.

## Benefits:

• Antioxydant agent

• Lower Cholesterol

• Improve Circulation

• Control Diabetes

## NUTRITIONAL RATIO

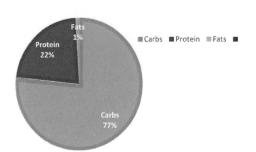

■Carbs ■Protein ■Fats ■

### Nutrition Values for 100g

**Energy:** 72 Kcal

**Carbohydrate:** 16.80 g

**Protein:** 2.50 g

**Total fat:** 0.10 g

| Vitamin | Value | RDA % |
|---|---|---|
| Vitamin A | 1190 IU | 35% |
| Vitamin C | 8 mg | 13% |
| Folates | 34 µg | 9% |
| Niancin | 0.200 mg | 1.5% |
| Pantothenic acid | 0.290 mg | 6% |
| Pyridoxine | 0.345 mg | 26.5% |
| Riboflavin | 0.020 mg | 2% |
| Thiamin | 0..060 mg | 5% |

| Minerals | Value | RDA% |
|---|---|---|
| Calcium | 37 mg | 4% |
| Copper | 0.088 mg | 10% |
| Iron | 1.20 mg | 15% |
| Magnesium | 21 mg | 5% |
| Manganese | 0.292 mg | 13% |
| Phosphorus | 60 mg | 8.5% |
| Selenium | 1.2 µg | 2% |
| Zinc | 0.40 mg | 4% |

# *Snow Peas*

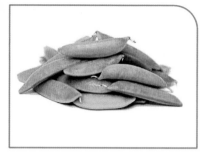

### How to store?

Refrigerate unwashed covered for up to 3 days.

### Benefits:

- Control blood sugar levels
- Prevents cancer
- Inprove digestion
- Boost immune System
- Improve vision

## NUTRITIONAL RATIO

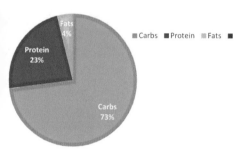

Carbs ■ Protein ■ Fats ■

### Nutrition Values for 100g

**Energy:** 81 Kcal

**Carbohydrate:** 14.45 g

**Protein:** 5.42 g

**Total fat:** 0.40 g

**Dietary fiber:** 5.1 g

| Vitamin | Value | RDA % |
|---|---|---|
| Vitamin A | 765 IU | 25.5% |
| Vitamin C | 40 mg | 67% |
| Vitamin E | 0.13 mg | 1% |
| Vitamin K | 24.8 µg | 21% |
| Folates | 65 µg | 16% |
| Niancin | 2.090 mg | 13% |
| Pantothenic acid | 0.104 mg | 2% |
| Pyridoxine | 0.169 mg | 13% |
| Riboflavin | 0.132 mg | 10% |
| Thiamin | 0.266 mg | 22% |

| Minerals | Value | RDA% |
|---|---|---|
| Calcium | 25 mg | 2.5% |
| Copper | 0.176 mg | 20% |
| Iron | 1.47 mg | 18% |
| Magnesium | 33 mg | 8% |
| Manganese | 0.410 mg | 18% |
| Selenium | 1.8 | 3% |
| Zinc | 1.24 mg | 11% |

# *Sorrel (Dock)*

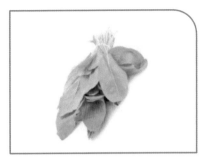

## How to store?

Sorrel is best used soon after purchase. If stored, store in a plastic bag, unwashed in the crisper section of the refrigerator for up to 3 days.

## Benefits:

- Aids in Digestion
- Improves Eyesight
- Regulates Blood Pressure
- Boosts Immunity

## NUTRITIONAL RATIO

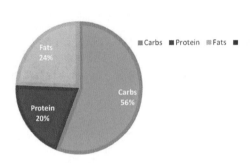

Carbs  Protein  Fats

Fats 24%
Carbs 56%
Protein 20%

### Nutrition Values for 100g

**Energy:** 22 Kcal

**Carbohydrate:** 3.20 g

**Protein:** 2.00 g

**Total fat:** 0.7 g

**Dietary fiber:** 2.9 g

| Vitamin | Value | RDA % |
|---|---|---|
| Vitamin A | 4000 IU | 133% |
| Vitamin C | 48 mg | 80% |
| Folates | 13 µg | 4% |
| Niancin | 0.500 mg | 3% |
| Pantothenic acid | 0.041 mg | 1% |
| Pyridoxine | 0.122 mg | 9% |
| Riboflavin | 0.100 mg | 8% |
| Thiamin | 0..040 mg | 3% |

| Minerals | Value | RDA% |
|---|---|---|
| Calcium | 44 mg | 4% |
| Copper | 0.131 mg | 14% |
| Iron | 2.40 mg | 30% |
| Magnesium | 103 mg | 26% |
| Manganese | 0.349 mg | 21% |
| Zinc | 0.20 mg | 2% |

# *Spaghetti Squash*

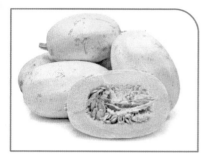

### How to store?

Store in a cool, well ventilated dry spot for up to a month.

### Benefits:

- Strengthens Bones
- Protects Heart Health
- Prevents Infections
- Improves Vision
- Improves Lung Health

## NUTRITIONAL RATIO

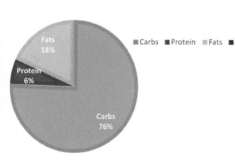

■ Carbs ■ Protein ■ Fats ■

## Nutrition Values for 100g

**Energy:** 31 Kcal

**Carbohydrate:** 6.91 g

**Protein:** 0.64 g

**Total fat:** 0.57 g

**Dietary fiber:** 1.5 g

| Vitamin | Value | RDA % |
|---|---|---|
| Vitamin A | 120 IU | 97% |
| Vitamin C | 2.1 mg | 70.5% |
| Folates | 12 µg | 21% |
| Niancin | 0.950 mg | 4% |
| Pantothenic acid | 0.360 mg | 1% |
| Pyridoxine | 0.101 mg | 15% |
| Riboflavin | 0.018 mg | 12% |
| Thiamin | 0.037 mg | 2% |

| Minerals | Value | RDA% |
|---|---|---|
| Calcium | 23 mg | 2% |
| Copper | 0.037 mg | 4% |
| Iron | 0.31 mg | 4% |
| Magnesium | 12 mg | 3% |
| Manganese | 0.125 mg | 0.5% |
| Phosphorus | 12 mg | 2% |
| Selenium | 0.3 µg | <0.5% |
| Zinc | 0.19 mg | 1.5% |

# *Spinach*

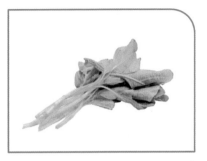

### How to store?

Discard yellow or damaged leaves. Remove stems and ribs if desired. Rinse in cold water, drain, wrap in paper towel. Cover, refrigerate two to four days. If in a bag, store as is.

### Benefits:

- Improves Eyesight
- Maintains Blood Pressure
- Strengthens Muscles
- Acts as Anti-ulcerative

## NUTRITIONAL RATIO

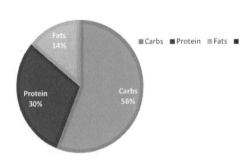

■ Carbs ■ Protein ■ Fats ■

### Nutrition Values for 100g

**Energy:** 23 Kcal

**Carbohydrate:** 3.63 g

**Protein:** 2.86 g

**Total fat:** 0.39 g

**Dietary fiber:** 2.2 g

| Vitamin | Value | RDA % |
|---------|-------|-------|
| Vitamin A | 9377 IU | 312% |
| Vitamin C | 28.1 mg | 47% |
| Vitamin E | 2.03 mg | 13.5% |
| Vitamin K | 482.9 µg | 402% |
| Folates | 194 µg | 48.5% |
| Niacin | 0.724 mg | 4.5% |
| Pantothenic acid | 0.065 mg | 1% |
| Pyridoxine | 0.195 mg | 15% |
| Riboflavin | 0.189 mg | 14.5% |
| Thiamin | 0..078 mg | 6.5% |

| Minerals | Value | RDA% |
|----------|-------|------|
| Calcium | 99 mg | 10% |
| Copper | 0.130 mg | 14% |
| Iron | 2.71 mg | 34% |
| Magnesium | 79 mg | 20% |
| Manganese | 0.897 mg | 39% |
| Zinc | 0.53 mg | 5% |

# Squash (Butternut)

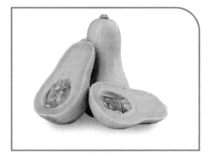

### How to store?

Keep in a cool, dry, dark and ventilated place for up to two months or at room temperature for one week. If cut, cover refrigerate for up to five days.

### Benefits:

- Antioxydant agent
- Improves Circulation
- Inprove digestion
- Prevents Birth Defects

## NUTRITIONAL RATIO

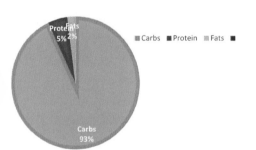

■ Carbs ■ Protein ■ Fats ■

### Nutrition Values for 100g

**Energy:** 45 Kcal

**Carbohydrate:** 11.69 g

**Protein:** 1.0 g

**Total fat:** 0.1 g

**Dietary fiber:** 2 g

| Vitamin | Value | RDA % |
|---|---|---|
| Vitamin A | 10630 IU | 354% |
| Vitamin C | 21 mg | 35% |
| Vitamin E | 1.44 mg | 10% |
| Vitamin K | 1.1 µg | 1% |
| Folates | 27 µg | 7% |
| Niancin | 1.200 mg | 8% |
| Pantothenic acid | 0.400 mg | 8% |
| Pyridoxine | 0.154 mg | 12% |
| Riboflavin | 0.020 mg | 2% |
| Thiamin | 0.100 mg | 8% |

| Minerals | Value | RDA% |
|---|---|---|
| Calcium | 48 mg | 5% |
| Copper | 0.072 mg | 8% |
| Iron | 0.70 mg | 9% |
| Magnesium | 34 mg | 9% |
| Manganese | 0.202 mg | 1% |
| Phosphorus | 33 mg | 5% |
| Selenium | 0.5 µg | <1% |
| Zinc | 0.15 mg | 1% |

# *Sugar Snap Peas*

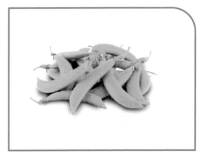

## How to store?

Sugar snap peas can be stored for up to a week in a sealed plastic bag in the refrigerator. Frozen peas can be stored in the freezer for up to 3 months.

## Benefits:

- Control blood sugar levels
- Prevents cancer
- Inprove digestion
- Boost immune

## NUTRITIONAL RATIO

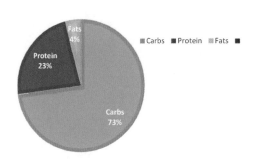

■ Carbs ■ Protein ■ Fats ■

Fats 4%
Protein 23%
Carbs 73%

### Nutrition Values for 100g

**Energy:** 42 Kcal

**Carbohydrate:** 7.55 g

**Protein:** 2.80 g

**Total fat:** 0.20 g

**Dietary fiber:** 2.6 g

| Vitamin | Value | RDA % |
|---|---|---|
| Vitamin A | 1087 IU | 36% |
| Vitamin C | 60 mg | 100% |
| Vitamin E | 39 mg | 2.5% |
| Vitamin K | 25 µg | 21% |
| Folates | 42 µg | 10.5% |
| Niancin | 0.600 mg | 4% |
| Pantothenic acid | 0.750 mg | 15% |
| Pyridoxine | 0.160 mg | 12% |
| Riboflavin | 0.080 mg | 6% |
| Thiamin | 0.150 mg | 12.5% |

| Minerals | Value | RDA% |
|---|---|---|
| Calcium | 43 mg | 4% |
| Copper | 0.079 mg | 9% |
| Iron | 2.08 mg | 26% |
| Magnesium | 24 mg | 6% |
| Manganese | 0.244 mg | 10.5% |
| Selenium | 0.7 µg | 1% |
| Zinc | 0.27 mg | 2% |

# *Sweet Potatoes*

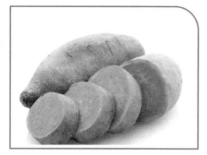

### How to store?

Keep uncovered at room temperature for up to 1 week.

### Benefits:

- Treat Inflammation
- Reduce Arthritis Pain
- Prevent Dehydration
- Relieve Asthma
- Treat Bronchitis
- Treat Stomach Ulcers

## NUTRITIONAL RATIO

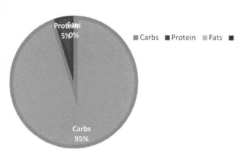

Proteins 5% 0%
Carbs 95%

■ Carbs  ■ Protein  ■ Fats  ■

### Nutrition Values for 100g

**Energy:** 86 Kcal

**Carbohydrate:** 20.12 g

**Protein:** 1.6 g

**Total fat:** 0.05 g

**Dietary fiber:** 3 g

| Vitamin | Value | RDA % |
|---|---|---|
| Vitamin A | 14.187 IU | 473% |
| Vitamin C | 2.4 mg | 4% |
| Vitamin E | 0.26 mg | 2% |
| Vitamin K | 1.8 µg | 1.5% |
| Folates | 11 µg | 3% |
| Niancin | 0.557 mg | 3.5% |
| Pantothenic acid | 0.80 mg | 16% |
| Pyridoxine | 0.209 mg | 15% |
| Riboflavin | 0.061 mg | 5.5% |
| Thiamin | 0..078 mg | 6.5% |

| Minerals | Value | RDA% |
|---|---|---|
| Calcium | 30 mg | 3% |
| Iron | 0.61 mg | 7.5% |
| Magnesium | 25 mg | 6% |
| Manganese | 0.258 mg | 11% |
| Phosphorus | 47 mg | 7% |
| Zinc | 0.30 mg | 3% |

# *Swiss Chard*

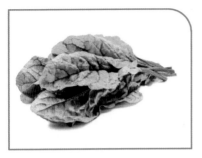

### How to store?

Store unwashed leaves in plastic bags in the crisper in the refrigerator for 2 to 3 days.

### Benefits:

- Brain Booster
- reduce blood pressure
- Reduce risk of diabetes
- Prevent colon cancer
- Eye care

## NUTRITIONAL RATIO

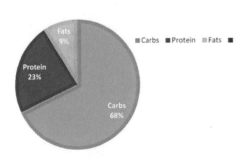

■ Carbs ■ Protein ■ Fats ■

### Nutrition Values for 100g

**Energy:** 19 Kcal

**Carbohydrate:** 3.74 g

**Protein:** 3.27 g

**Total fat:** 0.20 g

**Dietary fiber:** 1.6 g

| Vitamin | Value | RDA % |
|---|---|---|
| Vitamin A | 6116 IU | 204% |
| Vitamin C | 30 mg | 50% |
| Vitamin E | 1.89 mg | 12.5% |
| Vitamin K | 830 µg | 692% |
| Folates | 14 µg | 4.5% |
| Niacin | 0.400 mg | 2% |
| Pantothenic acid | 0.172 mg | 3% |
| Pyridoxine | 0.99 mg | 7.5% |
| Riboflavin | 0.090 mg | 7% |
| Thiamin | 0..040 mg | 3% |

| Minerals | Value | RDA% |
|---|---|---|
| Calcium | 51 mg | 5% |
| Copper | 0.179 mg | 20% |
| Iron | 1.80 mg | 22.5% |
| Magnesium | 81 mg | 20% |
| Manganese | 0.366 mg | 16% |
| Phosphorus | 46 mg | 6% |
| Selenium | 0.9 µg | 1.5% |
| Zinc | 0.39 mg | 3% |

# *Tomatillo*

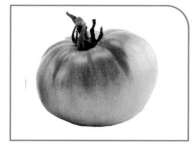

### How to store?

Refrigerate tomatillos loose or in an open container in the crisper drawer for 2-3 weeks.

### Benefits:

- Improve Vision
- Inprove digestion
- Boost Immune System
- Prevent lung & oral cancer
- Help in Weight Loss

## NUTRITIONAL RATIO

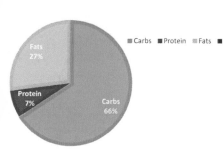

Carbs | Protein | Fats

### Nutrition Values for 100g

**Energy:** 32 Kcal

**Carbohydrate:** 5.84 g

**Protein:** 0.96 g

**Total fat:** 1.02 g

**Dietary fiber:** 1.9 g

| Vitamin | Value | RDA % |
|---------|-------|-------|
| Vitamin A | 114 IU | 4% |
| Vitamin C | 11.7 mg | 20% |
| Vitamin E | 0.38 mg | 2% |
| Vitamin K | 10.1 µg | 8.5% |
| Folates | 7 µg | 2% |
| Niancin | 0.1850 mg | 11.5% |
| Pyridoxine | 0.056 mg | 4% |
| Thiamin | 0..044 mg | 4% |

| Minerals | Value | RDA% |
|----------|-------|------|
| Calcium | 7 mg | 1% |
| Copper | 0.079 mg | 10% |
| Iron | 0.62 mg | 8% |
| Magnesium | 20 mg | 5% |
| Manganese | 0.153 mg | 6.5% |
| Phosphorus | 39 mg | 5.5% |
| Selenium | 0.5 µg | 1% |
| Zinc | 0.22 mg | 2% |

# *Tomato*

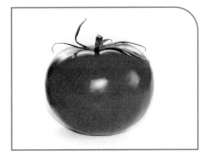

## How to store?

Keep tomatoes unwashed and uncovered at room temperature, out of direct sunlight, for up to one week. Do not refrigerate unless very ripe. To ripen, store in a paper bag at room temperature.

## Benefits:

- Antioxydant agent
- Protect the Heart
- Aid in Digestion
- Skin Care

## NUTRITIONAL RATIO

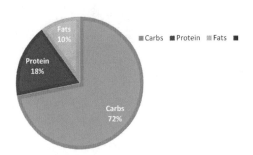

■ Carbs  ■ Protein  ▨ Fats  ■

Fats 10%
Protein 18%
Carbs 72%

### Nutrition Values for 100g

**Energy:** 18 Kcal

**Carbohydrate:** 3.9 g

**Protein:** 0.9 g

**Total fat:** 0.2 g

**Dietary fiber:** 3 g

| Vitamin | Value | RDA % |
|---|---|---|
| Vitamin A | 833 IU | 28% |
| Vitamin C | 13 mg | 21.5% |
| Vitamin E | 0.54 mg | 4% |
| Vitamin K | 7.9 µg | 6.5% |
| Folates | 15 µg | 4% |
| Niancin | 0.594 mg | 4% |
| Pyridoxine | 0.080 mg | 6% |
| Thiamin | 0..037 mg | 3% |

| Minerals | Value | RDA% |
|---|---|---|
| Calcium | 10 mg | 1% |
| Iron | 0.3 mg | 4% |
| Magnesium | 11 mg | 3% |
| Manganese | 0.15 mg | 6.5% |
| Phosphorus | 24 mg | 3% |
| Zinc | 0.17 mg | 1.5% |

# *Turnip*

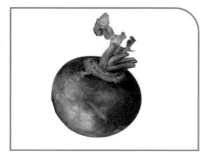

### How to store?

Store turnips in the refrigerator in a plastic bag for only a few days as they get bitter with prolonged storage.

### Benefits:

- Aid in Digestion
- Improve Blood Circulation
- Improve Heart Health
- Fight Inflammation
- Boost Metabolism

## NUTRITIONAL RATIO

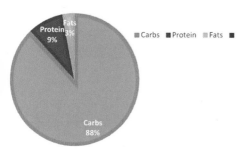

Carbs ■ Protein ■ Fats ■

## Nutrition Values for 100g

**Energy:** 28 Kcal

**Carbohydrate:** 6.43 g

**Protein:** 0.90 g

**Total fat:** 0.10 g

**Dietary fiber:** 1.8 g

| Vitamin | Value | RDA % |
|---|---|---|
| Vitamin A | 0 IU | 0% |
| Vitamin C | 21 mg | 35% |
| Vitamin E | 0.03 mg | <1% |
| Vitamin K | 0.1 µg | <1% |
| Folates | 15 µg | 4% |
| Niacin | 0.400 mg | 2.5% |
| Pantothenic acid | 0.200 mg | 4% |
| Pyridoxine | 0.090 mg | 7% |
| Riboflavin | 0.030 mg | 2.5% |
| Thiamin | 0..040 mg | 4% |

| Minerals | Value | RDA% |
|---|---|---|
| Calcium | 30 mg | 3% |
| Copper | 0.085 mg | 9% |
| Iron | 0.30 mg | 4% |
| Magnesium | 11 mg | 2.5% |
| Manganese | 0.134 mg | 6% |
| Zinc | 0.27 mg | 2% |

# *Watercress*

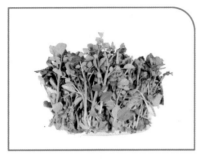

## How to store?

Rinse cut stems, blot with a paper towel and refrigerate in a plastic bag. Use within 4-5 days.

## Benefits:

- Prevents Breast Cancer
- Acts as Antidepressant
- Prevents Cognitive Disorders
- Prevents Stroke
- Improves Functioning of Thyroid Gland

## NUTRITIONAL RATIO

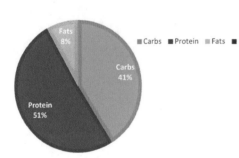

■ Carbs ■ Protein ■ Fats ■

Fats 8%
Carbs 41%
Protein 51%

### Nutrition Values for 100g

**Energy:** 11 Kcal

**Carbohydrate:** 1.29 g

**Protein:** 2.30 g

**Total fat:** 0.10 g

**Dietary fiber:** 0.5 g

| Vitamin | Value | RDA % |
|---|---|---|
| Vitamin A | 3191 IU | 106% |
| Vitamin C | 43 mg | 72% |
| Vitamin E | 1.0 mg | 7% |
| Vitamin K | 250 µg | 208% |
| Folates | 9 µg | 2% |
| Niancin | 0.200 mg | 6% |
| Pantothenic acid | 0.310 mg | 1% |
| Pyridoxine | 0.129 mg | 10% |
| Riboflavin | 0.120 mg | 9% |
| Thiamin | 0..090 mg | 7.5% |

| Minerals | Value | RDA% |
|---|---|---|
| Calcium | 120 mg | 12% |
| Copper | 0.077 mg | 8.5% |
| Iron | 0.20 mg | 2.5% |
| Magnesium | 21 mg | 5% |
| Manganese | 0.244 mg | 11% |
| Phosphorus | 60 mg | 8% |
| Selenium | 0.9 µg | 1.5% |
| Zinc | 0.11 mg | 1% |

# *Yam Root*

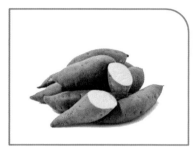

### How to store?

Store in a cool, dark place away from extreme temperatures. Yams will stay fresh for up to 10 days. Do not store in bags.

### Benefits:

- Lower bad cholesterol
- Low in sodium
- Prevent colon cancer
- Reduce cnstipation

## NUTRITIONAL RATIO

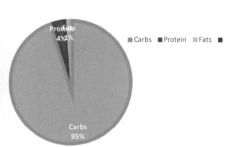

Carbs  Protein  Fats

### Nutrition Values for 100g

**Energy:** 108 Kcal

**Carbohydrate:** 27.88 g

**Protein:** 1.53 g

**Total fat:** 0.17 g

**Dietary fiber:** 4.1 g

| Vitamin | Value | RDA % |
|---|---|---|
| Vitamin A | 138 IU | 5% |
| Vitamin C | 17.1 mg | 28.5% |
| Vitamin E | 0.35 mg | 2% |
| Vitamin K | 2.3 µg | 2% |
| Folates | 23 µg | 6% |
| Niancin | 0.552 mg | 3.5% |
| Pantothenic acid | 0.314 mg | 7% |
| Pyridoxine | 0.293 mg | 23% |
| Riboflavin | 0.032 mg | 2.5% |
| Thiamin | 0.112 mg | 9.5% |

| Minerals | Value | RDA% |
|---|---|---|
| Calcium | 17 mg | 2% |
| Copper | 0.178 mg | 20% |
| Iron | 0.54 mg | 7% |
| Magnesium | 21 mg | 5% |
| Manganese | 0.397 mg | 17% |
| Phosphorus | 55 mg | 8% |
| Selenium | 0.7 µg | 0.5% |
| Zinc | 0.24 mg | 2% |

# *Zucchini*

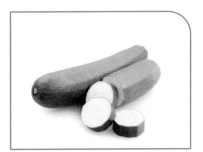

**How to store?**

Cover, refrigerate unwashed for up to one week.

**Benefits:**

- Slow down aging
- help lower cholesterol
- Improve eye health
- Lower blood pressure
- Enhance digestion

## NUTRITIONAL RATIO

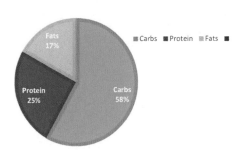

Carbs ■ Protein ■ Fats ■

Fats 17%
Protein 25%
Carbs 58%

### Nutrition Values for 100g

**Energy:** 17 Kcal

**Carbohydrate:** 3.11 g

**Protein:** 1.21 g

**Total fat:** 0.32 g

**Dietary fiber:** 1 g

| Vitamin | Value | RDA % |
|---|---|---|
| Vitamin A | 200 IU | 7% |
| Vitamin C | 17.9 mg | 30% |
| Vitamin E | 0.12 µg | 1% |
| Vitamin K | 4.3 µg | 4% |
| Folates | 24 µg | 6% |
| Niancin | 0.451 mg | 3% |
| Pantothenic acid | 0.204 mg | 5% |
| Pyridoxine | 0.163 mg | 13% |
| Riboflavin | 0.094 mg | 7% |
| Thiamin | 0..045 mg | 4% |

| Minerals | Value | RDA% |
|---|---|---|
| Calcium | 16 mg | 1.6% |
| Iron | 0.37 mg | 5% |
| Magnesium | 18 mg | 4% |
| Manganese | 0.177 mg | 8% |
| Phosphorus | 38 mg | 5% |
| Selenium | 0.2 µg | ≤1% |
| Zinc | 0.32 mg | 3% |